Using Health Data

Applying Technology to Work Smarter

Heather Grain &
Paula Procter

with contributions by Carol Bond

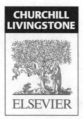

CHURCHILL
LIVINGSTONE

ELSEVIER

Sydney Edinburgh London New York Philadelphia St Louis Toronto

ELSEVIER

Churchill Livingstone
is an imprint of Elsevier

Elsevier Australia. ACN 001 002 357
(a division of Reed International Books Australia Pty Ltd)
Tower 1, 475 Victoria Avenue, Chatswood, NSW 2067

National Library of Australia Cataloguing-in-Publication Data

Grain, Heather.
Using health data : applying technology to work smarter / Heather Grain, Paula Procter.

ISBN: 978 0 7295 3889 3 (pbk.)

Includes index.
Bibliography.

Medical care.
Electronic data processing.
Information resources management.
Medical records--Data processing.

Procter, Paula.

651.504261

Publisher: Luisa Cecotti
Developmental Editor: Sabrina Chew
Publishing Services Manager: Helena Klijn
Editorial Coordinator: Lauren Allsop
Edited by Teresa McIntyre
Proofread by Matt Davies
Cover and internal design by saso content & design pty ltd
Typeset by Pindar New Zealand
Index by Michael Ferreira
Printed in Australia by Ligare

Using
Health
Data

Contents

This symbol indicates where material has been supplied for you on the CD.

The companion CD includes completed examples for each exercise so that you can check your progress.

Preface

The main challenge so far in the 21st century appears to be how to stay in control of our own information, and information we deal with as part of professional and personal lives. We can receive world news into our homes 24 hours a day, world successes and world tragedies are delivered in real time anywhere in the world, we have the option to be contactable 24 hours a day, seven days a week through mobile communications technology in any country, and we have the possibility of taking with us all of our favourite movies, audio and still images anywhere we go on a very small handheld device.

Healthcare is no different, and is rapidly developing technologies to support information acquisition, storage and retrieval around care as well as developing technologies for care itself, such as DNA-specific drug prescribing and nanotechnologies for smart homes. Those of us involved within or on the edge of healthcare and social care need to ensure that we are able to use the advancing information and communication technologies to support our delivery and evaluation of care for the benefit of those in our care, their relatives and their friends.

Due to the fact that we live in different hemispheres, we had to manage our writing process via the telephone, email and file sharing. We found it brought a new definition to team working: members who take virtual working to its limits. In today's healthcare systems, virtual teamwork is slowly dominating the working environment. Teleconferences via the Internet, transferring of documents virtually, and even working on documents through Web meetings are replacing the conventional methods.

This book represents a good starting point for those wanting to know more than just which button to press to fill in some data. We hope that you will find it of help and that you can use what you have learnt in your role successfully for patient/client benefit.

Heather Llewelyn Grain
Paula M Procter

Heather and I would like to dedicate this book to a dear friend, colleague and the person who first suggested the need for such a publication: Dr Moya Conrick. Sadly, Moya died before the writing really started; we hope she would have approved of our attempt to take her ideas forward and the end result which you see today. Both Heather and I would have welcomed her mentorship and input during the writing of the book, as well as her warmth and kindness and true Australian sense of humour when times got tough, but we had to resort to memories to bring us through, and what good memories those are.

Paula M Procter

Heather Llewelyn Grain, ADip MRA, GD DP, MHI, RMRA, FACHI
Director, Llewelyn Grain Informatics
Health Informatics – China Health Program, La Trobe University, Australia
Academic Fellow, Austin Health
Secretary and Fellow, Australian College of Health Informatics

Paula M Procter, RN, Cert Ed(FE), MSc, FBCS, CITP
Reader in Informatics and Telematics in Nursing, Faculty of Health and Wellbeing, Sheffield Hallam University, England
UK representative, International Medical Informatics Association – Nursing Informatics
Chartered IT Professional, British Computer Society
Board Member, NHS Faculty of Health Informatics

Carol Bond, EdD, MSc, RN, FBCS, CITP
Senior Lecturer, Health Informatics, School of Health and Social Care, Bournemouth University, England

Reviewers

Janice Lewis, DBA, MBus, BSc, FACHSE
Program Leader, Health Policy and Management Programs
School of Public Health, Curtin University of Technology, Australia

Keith Ward, BSc(H), DPSN, SRN, RMN, RNT
National Teaching Fellow and Principal Lecturer
School of Human and Health Sciences, University of Huddersfield, England

Sue Whetton, BA, DipT(P), Dip Cont Ed, MIS
Lecturer (Online Educational Development), Department of Rural Health
University of Tasmania, Australia

Janie Peterson, RN, BN, MEd (Adult), IC Cert
Lecturer and Director, Clinical Practice Based Learning
Recipient of 2008 Vice Chancellor's Citation for Outstanding Contributions
    to Student Learning
School of Health and Human Sciences, Southern Cross University, Australia

1 Introduction

1.1 Health information today

Healthcare is a social, scientific and information-based service. In today's world, health information is frequently collected, reported, delivered and processed by technology.

This book is designed to assist healthcare professionals of all types to understand the principles and processes for handling data in the electronic world. This book is not about making healthcare professionals into computer professionals – quite the reverse. It is about giving healthcare professionals the skills to apply their health expertise to greatest advantage and to retain control of the information they need to do their jobs. We believe that in order to deliver safe and effective healthcare and to manage health services today, all healthcare professionals, managers and carers as well as patients need to understand the basics of using health data and to some extent the systems that provide that information.

This book addresses the enduring problems faced by most healthcare professionals: how to collect health information in a way that is reliable; how to retrieve and transform that data into meaningful and accessible information once they have it; and how to present it for maximum effect.

This text provides detailed instructions and examples on the processes for retrieving and managing health data, along with practical health examples. Computer files containing data are also provided so that the skills highlighted in the text may be practised. Some basic statistical concepts are included along with relevant health examples. Note that while these data files include data which is consistent with common health data formats, they do not contain real patient data – they are fictitious.

1.1.1 Electronic health record initiatives

In the UK there are major developments involving information and communications technologies and healthcare. The government is spending over 12 billion pounds on health information developments.[1] This process is also occurring in other countries: the USA has introduced a national approach to sharing health information,[2] Canada has the Canada Health Infoway project,[3] and Australia the National E-Health Transition Authority.[4] There is great concern about to how to get healthcare professionals and the health information manager or healthcare manager involved in these projects. This book provides a practical entry point to knowledge on health information and how to collect and use it.

1.1.2   Relationship between this book and health informatics

Health informatics is the combination of computer science, information science and health science designed to assist in the management and processing of data, information and knowledge to support healthcare and healthcare delivery.[5]

As computer science has evolved, software products have become more standardised and offer users a much more extensive range of options and functionality. These days software you purchase is delivered as 'plug and play': just load it into your computer or download it from the Internet, and it installs and works for you straight off. The tasks performed by this complex and highly developed software have been predetermined by computer software engineers, in consultation with product users. Responsibility for software product development has rested largely with the information technology (IT) and information systems (IS) professionals. This often occurs because we, the users, have not understood either the potential of the technology or seen the opportunity to improve through change. For this reason, early software developments were often automated versions of the manual environment, forms and/or manual processes. For example, with an accounting package the rules for accounting have been long established, and local variations are managed by the provision of a set of local implementation rules for the software to apply.

When computers were first introduced into healthcare organisations in the 1970s most of the software was used to run administrative systems, such as patient billing, admission and discharge processing, and systems for statistical counting of services and diseases. There have been clinical uses of systems since the 1960s, but it is only in the past 10 years that the balance of systems ownership has increased the clinical impact. Only in the 1990s has software started to move significantly into the patient care environment, where it has the potential to broadly impact clinical practice. This change is difficult because of the complexity of health information and the fact that the systems necessary to support healthcare are more intricate, multidisciplinary and knowledge-dependent than are (much simpler) accounting or administrative systems. Difficulties arise from: the volume of information about each individual; the complexity of medical knowledge; and the highly integrated, multidisciplinary and multiorganisational nature of healthcare. Healthcare knowledge and practice has also changed significantly over the last 100 years – science has been applied throughout the practice of healthcare to improve patient outcomes, and these changes are ever more rapid and extensive.

In today's healthcare system, computers are increasingly the information storage and retrieval tool (the library, the note pad, the forms and the delivery system) for patient care. Now that this move into the clinical world has begun, it will not stop. The ball is rolling, and gaining momentum and size. What does this mean for healthcare? The move from paper-based to electronic mechanisms of information collection, storage and retrieval is a consistent, inevitable process and, as healthcare professionals responsible for patient care, it is vital for you to understand the data in your systems, and to control and make the most of this data. The benefits of this paradigm change accrue from the capacity to retrieve and distribute information more effectively in a computerised environment, and to provide access to clinical knowledge that is relevant to direct healthcare more quickly and effectively.

Would a doctor or nurse, or any other healthcare professional, allow an unqualified person to develop the work practices for patient care in the ward, surgery or consultation room? We would hope not! However, the application of computers in today's healthcare system has the potential to do just that. As computers have moved into the clinical world, many healthcare professionals are avoiding that understanding of the systems and data which is required to work in healthcare in the 21st century, believing that this is the role of IT staff. Health informatics links knowledge of healthcare requirements, processes, data, clinical capacity and safety to knowledge of the technology and system engineering. This combination allows healthcare professionals to ensure that systems are developed in a manner that: meets clinical needs and safety requirements; functions effectively with clinical workflow; and represents information in a way that supports clear meaning of clinical knowledge. These are tasks that can only be done by people with clinical expertise. In this way the clinician, health informatican and information professional function together to produce systems.

The proposition is not that clinical people become IT professionals – that would defeat the purpose. Rather, all clinical practitioners need to develop an understanding of the tools for data access and control for everyday support of healthcare, and to influence and control the systems introduced in their work environment. Health informaticans are most often healthcare professionals who have developed specialised knowledge in information systems and technology, although occasionally they have followed the opposite path as IT/IS professionals who have learnt about the requirements and specialisations of healthcare. These professionals plan, develop, implement and maintain clinical information systems and the infrastructure needed to allow these systems to function, such as computer-processable clinical terminology. Such systems include those for clinical decision support, direct care communication, order entry, clinical record keeping, knowledge management and the longer-established administrative and statistical systems. The profession has been recognised as a specialty – for example, recognition of Clinical Informatics as a specialty by the American Medical Association.

Whether using computerised or manual methods, the healthcare professional must be able to record and find information about individual patients and about health knowledge, and to inform themselves about the broader statistics and trends of health and healthcare within the bounds of information governance. Today this requires all healthcare professionals to have an understanding of computers. When you abrogate responsibility for health information systems in this emerging healthcare environment where clinical knowledge is provided by computer systems, you effectively give away your control of those systems. It isn't necessary or appropriate for healthcare professionals to have a detailed knowledge of exactly *how* these systems work – but we must contribute to the system operation process and ensure that this process is safe and appropriate. We also have a responsibility to take maximum advantage of the information available to us when treating patients.

This book focuses on a specific area of health informatics – data manipulation and presentation. As data is the core of healthcare provision this is an essential skill for all healthcare professionals, whether they envisage going on to a profession in health informatics or not. This book does not intend to make you a health informatics expert; rather, it aims to explain to health professionals:

- their responsibilities and opportunities when using health information systems
- what to do with data once it has been recorded
- how to ask questions of stored information
- how to improve data capture
- how to use the tools and processes available through computer software to maximise the value of the data collected
- what methods exist to improve the quality of the data collected in healthcare.

Example 1.1 – Clinical information changes

In patient care you collect information all the time (in manual and computer systems). Let's consider the manual system – where you write down some of the information, tell some of it to others with whom you work, and remember some of it. You apply the information in ways that are affected by your professional training, experience and expertise. The electronic environment doesn't change these principles, but it *does* change the where and how of information recording, how you can access clinical knowledge, and increases the range of analysis that can be made of processes.

The traditional clinical trial process is being challenged by new availability of clinical information. In the traditional research model, a hypothesis is generated that indicates an expected response to a given situation. In the information-rich healthcare environment that is emerging, sufficient information is available that common characteristics (treatments, patient profiles, combinations of drugs/ diseases) which present either positive or negative outcomes (compared with the norm) can be identified automatically – and trials of comparative cohorts can be identified using retrospective data. This process can reduce both the time needed to identify potential improvements or dangers in healthcare, and also the time required to implement these changes.

Computers are capable of providing best-practice information to support clinical care – but this process is completely dependent on the data stored in patients' computerised records and on the ability to represent that knowledge in a computer-processable way.

Example 1.2 – Reporting data changes

In the traditional healthcare structure there are strong departmental segregations of process and information. Each department, hospital and community centre reports data against specific programs and requirements. These data are often inconsistent with each other – counting similar or the same things in different ways.

Traditional collection systems often require manual collection of statistics or financial information for reporting, and extraction of data from manual records. These processes are also changing. There is an increasing desire – and the practical capacity – to automate reporting of data from the computer-based information systems used to collect data for patient care. This process is called secondary data use, or by-product data use. This does *not* mean that such use is less important than the primary patient care use, but that greater advantage and consistency of data is achieved by using that primary care data to automatically report to authorities. In this way, less effort is required to produce these reports and more effort can thus be put into direct patient care. Reporting is also more accurate and timely. The process has the potential for a far more integrated look at both patient care and the services provided across the whole spectrum of healthcare.

In each of these examples, data users have access to more extensive data than they would have had in the past, and have the capacity both to understand how that data could be used and to obtain that data themselves from the computer system (or to ask the information technology professionals to obtain specific data for them).

This book strongly advocates the inclusion of clinical and information technology professionals as team members to support the system and data requirements of healthcare professionals, the objective being that the healthcare professional retains responsibility for and governance of the system and for the data in that system.

1.2   Who should read this book

This book is for the 'doers' and 'users' of health data, rather than the IT professional (though they too are welcome to read it). If you are on the list below, or if you work with anyone on the list below – this book is for you:

- carer or patient
- doctor
- nurse
- dentist
- allied health professional

- traditional medicine practitioner
- health information manager
- health classification or terminologist
- health administrator
- health researcher
- epidemiologist
- IT/IS professional wishing to understand specific health data issues.

The approach of this book is practical, informative and accessible. It is based on 'real' examples from healthcare practice to illustrate, demonstrate and provide advice. It discusses the pitfalls and offers some resolutions, along with information on successful strategies to handle common issues. The book also addresses how data can be presented to gain the greatest benefit using various quantitative quality-control charting and plotting methods.

Through the exercises and information provided in this book, the reader is assisted in understanding how to transform qualitative data into quantitative measures, how to link data from multiple sources to create new information, and how to differentiate between different types of health data (e.g. administrative, for planning, for resource scheduling, clinical evidence).

1.2.1   What readers will gain from this book

Health data and the uses it has in supporting healthcare are unique to the healthcare sector. Tools exist which assist in the understanding and development of health data that are specific to the industry, and these tools will be explained.

After completing study of this book the reader should be able to:

- assess the quality of health data used for decision making or care
- design relevant data collection definitions
- extract data from existing data storage facilities
- define data required for reporting, research or other activities – to enable technical staff to extract data that is relevant to your needs quickly and effectively
- understand the potential of information systems to improve information availability
- manage available information and translate that information into usable formats to support decision making in healthcare
- decide which computer software tool/s are the most appropriate to manipulate data in a given situation
- decide the best format and design features to represent data accurately and 'tell the story' of the information.

1.2.2   Expected reader background

Although it is accepted that understanding and management of data are essential in healthcare, the literature and recent research in nursing[6] demonstrate that healthcare professionals lack education in basic computing. This situation is common throughout the healthcare professions, both clinical and administrative. For this reason this book does not assume computer knowledge beyond the basic. Our definition of basic comprises the following:

- use of a mouse (navigation, left-click, right-click and double-click)
- basic computer operations (turning it on and off, opening a document, running a program)
- searching the Internet
- using email.

There is no expectation that readers will know anything significant about hardware, and we will include some instruction on this – in so far as it affects the use of tools and data.

It is assumed that readers will be able to input data; if not, there are many 'pure' computer books that address this aspect of data collection. Local health software producers have their own procedure manuals – this book does not seek to explain the basics of IT nor of your local health software. It is generic to the management of health data in any environment.

1.3 How to use this book

Throughout this text we concentrate on the principles, supported by case-based examples using currently available software packages. The use of case-based examples will help to contextualise the data for the reader. The 'cases' used for the self-study exercises will move beyond the generally expected single-entity patient case; it is intended that the exercise may well be multifaceted and multifactorial to allow for interrelationships in terms of data and information extraction. Information is also interdisciplinary and often multidisciplinary.

The practical section of this book is divided into four chapters, each of which provides specific skills. Chapter 2, *About data*, covers principles of data entry and quality, storage and retrieval – basic elements that apply to all data in healthcare. We advise that this chapter and its associated exercises be completed before working on other chapters.

Following this, there are stand-alone chapters on presentation and sharing of data, and on spreadsheets and databases. The information provided on each individual data-management tool is self-sufficient – you don't need to read the database section if you only want to understand spreadsheets.

Each chapter contains examples of a data extraction or manipulation process, which are used to work through the steps of that process. You are given the opportunity to work these through alongside the text, then to try an exercise on your own. The companion CD includes completed examples for each exercise so that you can check your progress. This symbol indicates where material has been supplied for you on the CD:

Within each chapter the structure follows the same pattern:

- clear specification of the starting point in the example cases
- what each process does – a short description of the process
- why you would use it – explained through case-based examples that help you understand the relevance of the process
- the process principles – a generic, detailed explanation of what the process does
- a complete worked example of the process including screen shots that explain every step of the process
- an exercise for you to work through that covers the same principles of the process, for additional practice and understanding.

To gain maximum benefit from this book, it is important that you follow the complete process in each section by working through each example, and that you try the exercise. It is often simple to understand the process and objectives while you read them, but when confronted with making choices in front of the computer it can be much more difficult – it is for this reason that the authors have developed the exercises to support your practice. In this case practice really is the only route to confidence and understanding.

1.4   Some notes on software

The software discussed in this book is primarily Microsoft's Windows-based Office suite. We have chosen this because it is an integrated package widely in use in the healthcare system, and as such readers will likely be familiar with aspects of it. It is also the software most frequently available in the healthcare work environment and as such, the tool of convenience.

The fortunate position if you are using a 'suite' of applications is that once you have mastered the basic control commands for one application, you can often use those commands in the others. Also, it is often simple to transfer data between different applications within the suite. Having said this, the methods and principles we cover are generic and can be applied to other software packages. By and large, if you can do a certain thing in an Office program, then you will be able to do similar things in another software package such as found in Open Source solutions – it is simply a case of using the Help function to find out which keys to press.

We have chosen primarily to demonstrate the examples with Office 2007, as this is the most recent version, and many readers who are familiar with older versions will be making the transition as well as getting to know it from scratch. However, since many healthcare organisations will not yet have upgraded to the latest version, instructions are also included for Office 2003.

If you are using Office 2003, Word, PowerPoint, Access and Excel documents can all be opened using Office 2007; they are compatible with the newer version. This compatibility does not always work in the other direction. Now that Office 2007 is widely available, you may receive files created using this software. If you are using Office 2003, you may find that they will not open. In this case you will need to contact the originator of the document and ask them to save the file in Office 2003 format. Figure 1.1 shows the option to save a Word file in an older version; the principle is the same for PowerPoint and Excel. It is not possible to backwards-convert a database file with a simple action like this.

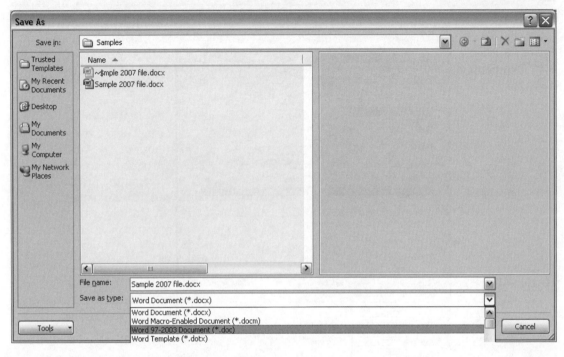

Figure 1.1 Saving a file as an earlier version of Office

The equivalent versions for Macintosh computers are Office 2008 and Office 2004, and they work in very similar ways to the Windows-based programs. It is perhaps just worth noting that Mac users with a single-click mouse can press **CTRL-click** to get the equivalent of a right-click in Windows.

1.4.1 Finding your way around

The important thing to note is that, by and large, the different versions of Office allow you to do the same things, but the *pathways* into the commands are different. So it's a matter of locating the command in your particular version. Don't be afraid to click the different tabs looking for what you want, and use your mouse to hover over icons to access explanatory information or submenus.

The **Page Layout** ribbon (Fig 1.2) contains the elements of page layout that you will want to change most often. Hover over an icon to get an explanation, and left-click on an icon to get a submenu to choose from.

Some submenus have a 'more options' or 'custom options' line at the bottom, and clicking on this will bring up a dialog box. Figure 1.3 shows the dialog box that comes up for Page Setup.

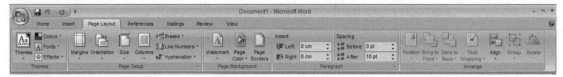

Figure 1.2 Page Layout ribbon in Word 2007

Figure 1.3 Word
2007 Page Setup
dialog box

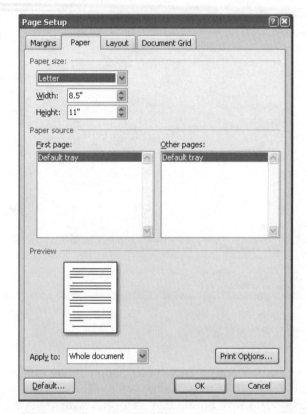

Alternatively, you can click on the little arrow to the right of **Page Setup** at the bottom of the Page Layout ribbon to bring up the same dialog box:

In Word 2003, instead of the tabs system there is a menu bar near the top of the window (Fig 1.4); left-click on one of the menu items to call up a submenu. Again, you can hover over any icon in the next bar down to get an explanation.

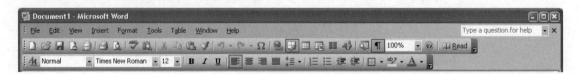

Figure 1.4 Menu bar in Word 2003

Notice the two down arrows at the bottom of the submenu (Fig 1.5) – this means that all the options on the menu are not currently being displayed. Either wait for them to come into view, or left-click the down arrows.

Office has built in a 'used often' function to the menus, and will always show the options that are most commonly used by you first. As you get used to this feature you will either love it or not.

Figure 1.5
Format submenu in Word 2003 – reduced version

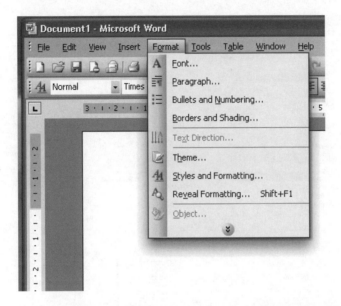

Figure 1.6
Format submenu in Word 2003 – full version

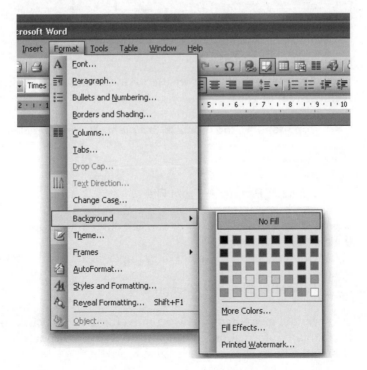

Note how hovering over the little black arrow on a menu item calls up a further submenu of choices.

In Word 2003, if you click on **File** in the main menu bar and choose **Page Setup** you will get the dialog box shown in Figure 1.7. Compare this with Figure 1.3 – you can see how Word 2007 and Word 2003 are similar behind the scenes (there is just an extra tab in the Word 2007 dialog box).

Figure 1.7 Page Setup dialog box in Word 2003

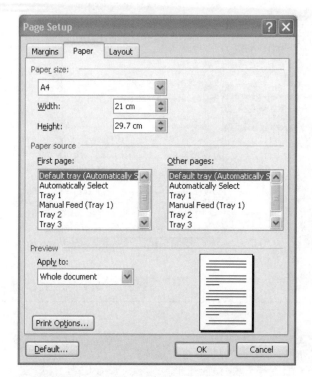

Describing menu choices

For Office 2003, the format we use for indicating where things are in the menu system is:

Top menu ➤ 2nd menu ➤ 3rd menu ➤ *file name (if any)*

For example:

Insert ➤ Picture ➤ From File . . . ➤

will open up a dialog box where you can enter a filename or browse to find the picture you need.

Often there is no filename. For example, in an Excel 2003 worksheet:

Format ➤ Sheet ➤ Background

gives you the menu item that is required for use – left-click to access Background information. When you are ready, return to the main screen by closing the dialog box using the 'x' at top right.

In Office 2007, the pathway is:

Home ➤ Font ➤ 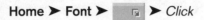 **➤** *Click*

– you click on the box arrow to access the Format Cells dialog box which includes a tab for Background.

EXERCISE 1.1

Take a few moments to explore the menus in the programs you use most often, to get a feel for where commands can be found.

1.4.2   Using the Help function

When you aren't sure how to do a particular function, or have trouble, a Help facility is provided. It is important to remember that to use Help effectively you need to know the words used to describe what you are trying to do, such as 'print' or 'make a table'. To open Help press the **F1** key at the top left-hand side of the keyboard, above the numbers row.

Figure 1.8 shows the common areas of Help (in Word 2007). If you click on any of these headings, detailed help will be provided (Fig 1.9). The more detailed screen provides information about common problems for that topic area, and also provides a search facility (near the top of the window) where you can enter a specific query.

Figure 1.8 Help headings in Word 2007

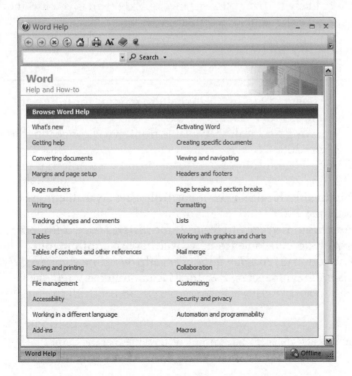

Figure 1.9
Detailed topic
subheadings in
Word Help

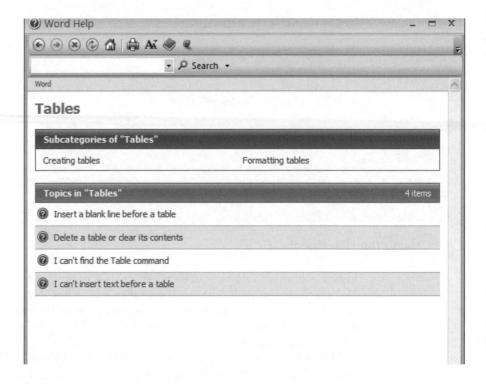

Use the information in this book to assist you if you request help – the terms used in the text will be terms the Help system 'understands' and it will be more likely to give you assistance quickly than if you use another word that may have the same or a similar meaning.

References

1. Department of Health, National Programme for Information Technology. London: HMSO, 2002.
2. Connecting for Health. Available from: www.connectingforhealth.org [12 June 2009].
3. Canada Health Infoway. Available from: www.infoway-inforoute.ca [12 June 2009].
4. National E-Health Transition Authority. Available from: www.nehta.gov.au [12 June 2009].
5. Australian College of Health Informatics, *Health Informatics: an introduction to the field*. Available from: www.achi.org.au/informatics [7 June 2009].
6. Lazakidou A, ed. *Handbook of research on informatics in healthcare and biomedicine*. Hershey, PA: Idea Group Reference, 2006.

2 About data

Learning objectives

When this chapter is completed you will be able to:
- understand the difference between data and information
- assess the likely quality of data being used
- understand the relevance of health data standards
- define an element of health data and access existing definitions
- understand the implications and considerations for ethical, secure use of data.

What *is* 'data'? What is all the fuss?

In the old manual world, we just wrote things on paper. Sometimes that paper had structure (i.e. forms) and sometimes not (i.e. lined blank paper). The more structured the format on completion, the easier it was to find the piece of information you wanted, provided the person who originally captured that information had put the right stuff in the right place.

This chapter covers: what we mean when we say *data*; how data are described; and some of the processes that can be used to improve the quality of that data. It is intended that this knowledge will develop your skills in the definition of data and in clinical information representation, so that you understand how to improve data collection systems, and know the potential and restrictions of data use.

You think you've just conquered your iPod or MP3 player or – even more challenging – your mobile phone, and along comes a new feature that makes your machine and your knowledge redundant. Although computer systems can often feel like this, as they do change rapidly, the data within them is not so variable.

2.1 What is data?

The detailed and complex area of healthcare requires the use of specific terminology. Information science is no different. Although you don't need to understand *all* the 'magic words' of computer science, there are advantages to understanding some of the more commonly used ones.

Data: 'Representation of real world facts, concepts or instructions in a formalized manner suitable for communication, interpretation or processing by human beings or by automatic means'.[1]

Examples of data are:

4
Black
Right leg
Pneumonia

It is important to note that data have no meaning until put into context. This is achieved by either relating one item of data to another, or by putting data into a 'field' or 'data element'.

Context	Data
Age at admission	4
Hair colour	Black
Site of wound	Right leg
Diagnosis	Pneumonia

Data element: 'The descriptive name of the information object that contains data. A unit of data for which the definition, identification, representation and permissible values are specified by means of a set of attributes'.[2]

Information is technically not the same as data. Information is defined as: 'data that are interpreted, organized and structured'.[3]

For example: *Mary Smith is four years old.* This is information that can be applied to an individual instance; it is something that is a fact about a given person or circumstance.

Level	Example
Data	4
Data element	Age at admission '4'
Data in a person's record (information about Mary)	Mary's record shows her 'Age at admission' to be '4'

Knowledge is more circumspect. Knowledge takes data about individuals and applies this more broadly in order to generally inform. The fact that one individual has a condition does not mean that you have knowledge about that condition in general. However, when you compare information about individuals over a period of time, comparing commonalities, you may gain general knowledge about that condition and how it occurs in the community.

Knowledge is defined as 'information that has been synthesized so that interrelationships are identified and formalized'.[3]

An example of such synthesis is the knowledge that children under five are more susceptible to influenza virus. This knowledge can be applied:

Mary is more susceptible to influenza virus than an adult would be.

Other common examples of knowledge include medical knowledge generated from evidence-based medical practice, such as the knowledge that smoking cigarettes is a risk factor for contracting throat cancer.

To use data in health systems with accuracy, one must understand both the item of data and how it is represented, and the data element within which it is stored. The way in which we capture and store data items has an affect upon their ability to be computer-processed and upon the quality of the data.

2.2 Quality issues

'More and more companies are discovering that data quality issues are causing large losses in money, time, and missed opportunities'.[4] Healthcare is no different. Healthcare is an information-based industry where there are vast quantities of data collected for a wide range of purposes. It is necessary to understand each purpose at the point of gathering, representing, storing, protecting and retrieving (using) that data if the data are to be accurately collected.

Issues of data quality include an awareness of data structure, codes and collection.

2.2.1 At the point of collection

The first issue is the collection of data. When information is collected, you need to make it easy for people to record data quickly and to allow correct information to be recorded.

Healthcare is not only information intensive, it is often highly stressful. Consider a triage nurse in an emergency department with a queue of people awaiting attention. The design of the information system can have an impact on what is recorded and on the accuracy of that information. Is the information relevant to the triage process and to that patient's immediate care? Is the information easy to record? These issues will affect the quality of the information recorded.

Some of the specific issues relevant to data collection are outlined overleaf. When selecting computer systems or designing, approving or commenting upon the suitability of systems or data, these issues should be considered and assessed.

Q Does the data cover all possibilities? Are you able to record the information that represents what has actually occurred?

Where the user can't represent the real world within the recording system, they will either leave information blank, or choose the closest option available (according to their perspective). These choices lead to less than accurate data collection.

Example 2.1

Clinical information must accurately represent the real-world information. When collecting information for reporting, epidemiology and statistical usage, information is often grouped so that like conditions are presented grouped together and represented by one code. This is not appropriate in the direct-care environment, where there is a necessity to represent the *detail* rather than the grouped generality. Figure 2.1 indicates how classifications group similar conditions. In particular, the classification of 'other specified disorders of thyroid' is one that is useful when counting and grouping clinical information – but of little value in the clinical environment.

Figure 2.1
An example of grouping of classifications

E07	Other disorders of thyroid
E07.0	Hypersecretion of calcitonin
	C-cell hyperplasia of thyroid
	Hypersecretion of thyrocalcitonin
E07.1	Dyshormogenetic goitre
	Familial dyshormogenetic goitre
	Pendred's syndrome
	Excludes transitory congenital goitre with normal function (P72.0)
E07.8	Other specified disorders of thyroid
	Abnormality of thyroid binding globulin

Q Can you record unknown values?

If the person recording information doesn't know, or can't find out, the information to enter into a specific data item, does the system allow them to record this?

There are many different types of unknown data. In some systems there is a desire to capture information about *why* data is unknown. For example:

- Have not asked (will require follow-up)
- Unable to collect (patient unconscious) (will require follow-up but not immediately)
- Patient would not provide details
- Patient could not provide details.

These are only some of the variations that can be useful in designing systems for collecting data. The single concept of 'unknown' is usually all that is needed when counting or statistically evaluating the data; the difference between that and the options outlined above is the clinical relevance and ability to understand the need for follow-up to improve (complete) the data collection. It is important that you are able to evaluate what type of data you are collecting and the way you intend to use the information.

Unknown values can be valuable to support follow-up. If you record that a value is unknown at admission, it is easy to develop a report of inpatients with unknown values (those unable to be collected or not asked) and to visit these patients to obtain details.

Is detail retained or lost? Q

The quality of data can be affected by loss of detail.

Example 2.2

If you collect information about place of birth at a country level, you lose detail about the state or territory in which patients were born. This makes the assumption that the more detailed information will never be needed. Twenty years ago we collected only at the country level; today we collect at both the country level and the state level for those born in Australia. The old data are less detailed than the current data, and therefore difficulties arise when considering the trends of that data over time.

The current trend towards Electronic Health Records requires the collection of more detailed information to support clinical needs; administrative data (such as place of birth) is also becoming more specific. Aggregation (grouping) of data for reporting purposes can often be done automatically by computer systems, thereby giving the option of reporting at the detailed level or the grouped level according to our needs.

2.2.2   The issue of relevance

To obtain accurate information, it is important to consider the *purpose* of the data collection and the *relevance* of the data to those collecting it. If data has value to those collecting it, they are likely to want it to be accurate and timely, and be prepared to take time and care when collecting it. To assess relevance of the data being collected you should ask:

- Is the data relevant to those who are collecting it?
- If the information is collected by nursing or clinical staff, is it of value to them?
- Is there a way of obtaining the information needed in a manner that would be of use to the data collectors?

How is the information used locally? For example, if the local system needs data on a patient's requirements for an interpreter, then this is likely to be accurately collected. However, some epidemiological collections wish to obtain information on the language spoken at home. This is a piece of information that has no local use in an inpatient setting, but may be of value to a district nurse – different data suit different needs and this must be borne in mind.

If you need to collect data that has no local relevance, it is important that you ensure that those collecting the data understand the importance of the data items and how they will be used outside of the collector's environment.

2.2.3   Raw data

Raw data is data exactly as it is captured, without modification or analysis. The quality of data throughout the information system will be affected by the capacity and motivation of the individual who enters the information into systems or forms.

Will the person who has to collect the information have access to the raw data? **Q**

Example 2.3

A form designed to collect information about patients attending a local emergency room included the data element 'Country of Birth'. In this emergency department the detail of country of birth is not of high clinical importance, and is often left blank on the form. When this form is later used for data entry into the computer system, the person responsible for the data entry does not have access to the patient, who has probably gone home.

If the data on the form is not correct, the clerical staff have no access to the original data – in this case the patient – so that they can find the correct information.

Is the data required for entry into the system able to be recorded accurately? Do the codes used allow all options to be recorded? **Q**

If data cannot be recorded accurately, with all options permitted, we get the problem of a 'best guess' being recorded. In this situation the data collected may misinterpret what was meant in the raw data.

Example 2.4

Clerical staff are required to enter the 'Country of Birth' into the system, but the person filling in the form has recorded *USSR*, a country that no longer exists. There are many possible countries within the former USSR that could be recorded in the system, and an assumption would thus have to be made about where the person was actually born.

Are there choices to be made in data entry? **Q**

Where there are choices to be made, it is important that the individual who collects the data understands the rules and intention of the collection in order to ensure that valid and relevant choices are made. The collector must understand *how* the information will be used, *by whom* and *for what purpose*.

Example 2.5 – Collection of 'Principal Diagnosis' data element

The diagnosis to be recorded in this field is defined as:

The diagnosis established after study to be chiefly responsible for occasioning an episode of admitted patient care, an episode of residential care or an attendance at the healthcare establishment.[5]

This definition was established by the Health Data Standards Committee, and is represented in Australia's national health metadata registry, METeOR.[6] It is important to recognise that this definition was *not* established to support clinical communication – it is not necessarily the condition that the treating doctor wants to tell the general practitioner about (the most important diagnosis at discharge), but must be recorded according to the national definition and statistical reporting requirements.

The principal diagnosis is collected at discharge, often on discharge or referral letters used to communicate with other healthcare providers such as the general practitioner who is responsible for the ongoing care of the patient. The disease condition of most relevance at that time is the one needing ongoing care. This presents two difficulties: first, the conflict in attempting to take clinical communication data and using that data as the basis for fiscal reporting and identification and analysis of public health disease trends; and second, that those who record and process the data that results from this collection must understand the potential issues in collection and the relationship between that and the quality of the data.

Interpreting other people's data without a clear understanding can lead to misinformation. In healthcare such problems often arise where clerical interpretation of clinical data is made; this occurs most frequently when data is extracted from clinical records. This is a particular concern when the person interpreting the clinical data is not trained in the terminology and clinical anatomy, physiology and pathology processes as well as the objectives and processes required for the rules of data collection.

Are there **Q** *agreed methods for making choices when interpreting raw data?*

The clearer the rules for making decisions about data to be collected, the more likely the data collected will be accurate. In the Australian healthcare system there are established rules for choices of principal diagnosis. These rules make a valuable contribution to accurate data collection and usage. Where such rules are not proscriptive and clear, choices made may vary and comparable data will not be obtained. Note that while these rules fit the purpose of data reporting, they would not necessarily be the rules to apply when preparing data for clinical communication.

> **Example 2.6**
>
> If a person is admitted to hospital for surgery for a condition, but is discharged without the surgery having been performed (perhaps because they have a head cold and are not a good surgical risk), the Australian national coding rules provide guidance on how this is to be handled:
>
> **Original treatment plan not carried out**
>
> *Sequence as the principal diagnosis the condition which after study occasioned the admission to the hospital, even though treatment may not have been carried out due to unforeseen circumstances (see also ACS 0011 Admission for surgery not performed).*[5]

2.2.4   Data quality improvement strategies

If you are designing procedures and systems to collect quality health information, the following strategies should be employed.

- *Collect meaningful data at source. Collect data that is of value to the people collecting it and that is understood by these people.*

Clinical staff need to communicate information about patient diagnosis at discharge. This information could be collected in a manner that suits clinical communication and purpose, and administrative decisions could be made (according to the secondary use purposes) to reorder the data to meet that need.

- *Data should be entered into the system directly at the point of capture rather than being passed through multiple people or forms, as each pass may change minor elements of the data or the meaning of that data.*

Rather than designing systems that require a form to be filled in for someone else to update patient details, completion of the update directly at the ward, or better still bedside, is more likely to reduce errors. Handheld devices are increasingly being used to support both information capture and information display in healthcare. These technical advances offer a great opportunity to give the clinical staff member better data, but also to reduce the reporting load (by reduction of forms and transfer of information manually to third parties) and improving the quality of data.

- *Design data collections to allow entry of accurate information (include unknown values). Include the capacity to collect free text when codes don't 'fit'.*

In this way a code can be chosen, acknowledged to be a 'best guess', and the textual real-world meaning can be stored. This not only improves the quality of data, but gives the opportunity to review and improve the coding system/s used. As healthcare moves to the use of electronic systems for the representation of clinical information, this approach is particularly important to ensure safe and accurate communication for clinical care.

- *Provide infrastructure that will support timely data collection.*

It is important that systems are designed to make it physically easy to collect information. This requires consideration of workflow and clinical process. Design systems to collect information in a manner that suits clinical procedures, and provide equipment to support data collection. In particular, consider the use of barcodes and other automated methods of obtaining accurate information in a quick and simple way. Handheld devices are increasingly being used as a mechanism to simplify the process of data entry and to allow data collection within appropriate clinical workflows.

- *Establish standard definitions for data items and data concepts.*

Ensure that all parties involved understand what information is required and agree upon what the information actually represents (definitions). Establish standard rules that make it clear what is to be collected where there are choices available.

There exist standards that are used to describe health data. The information used to describe and explain data is called *metadata*. The International Standard for metadata registries[7] provides a guideline for the definition of health data. Figure 2.2 on page 24 provides an example of metadata from the Australian Metadata Register (METeOR).[6] The use of openly available, agreed definitions and structures for data improve the consistency of information collection, support comparison and the use of information over time. Each data element, or field, is defined by a definition that clearly indicates the values used in the field at a given point in time and provides guidelines on the intended use of the data. The metadata also clearly indicate who is responsible for the definition of the data and the source of the information, thereby giving you the opportunity to contact the source if there are questions or issues related to the use of the information.

Cancer staging—staging basis of cancer, code A

Identifying and definitional attributes

Metadata item type:	Data Element
Short name:	Staging basis of cancer
METeOR identifier:	296981
Registration status:	Health, Standard 04/06/2004
Definition:	The timing and evidence for T, N and M cancer stage values, as represented by a code.
Data Element Concept:	Cancer staging—staging basis of cancer

Value domain attributes

Representational attributes

Representation class:	Code
Data type:	String
Format:	A
Maximum character length:	1
Permissible values:	Value Meaning
	P Pathological
	C Clinical

Collection and usage attributes

Guide for use: CODE P Pathological

Pathological stage is based on histological evidence acquired before treatment, supplemented or modified by additional evidence acquired from surgery and from pathological examination.

CODE C Clinical

Clinical stage is based on evidence obtained prior to treatment from physical examination, imaging, endoscopy, biopsy, surgical exploration or other relevant examinations.

Refer to the latest edition of the UICC reference manual TNM Classification of Malignant Tumours for coding rules.

Source and reference attributes

Submitting organisation: Australian Institute of Health and Welfare

Data element attributes

Collection and usage attributes

Collection methods: From information provided by the treating doctor and recorded on the patient's medical record.

Relational attributes

Implementation in Data Set Specifications:

Cancer (clinical) DSS Health, Superseded 07/12/2005
Cancer (clinical) DSS Health, Standard 07/12/2005
Cancer (clinical) DSS Health, Candidate 14/09/2006

Figure 2.2 Example of metadata

2.3 International standards

Clear meaning and representation of data is required if we want a computer to be able to manage and analyse that data. International standards exist that describe how to define data.[8] These standards are increasingly being used in healthcare as a mechanism to communicate, openly and broadly to the health community, the meaning and codes used to describe common items of data. Some countries have a coordinated standards-based approach to these data which have been published and made readily available.

The process of data development is described in this section. The principles for the development of quality consistent health data items include:

1 Creating or adopting data standards as part of data development.
2 Using national or international standards wherever available and applicable.
3 Ensuring that data development is system independent.
4 Making the purpose of the data collection clear.
5 Ensuring that data are fit for that purpose.
6 Continual improvement – data development may be incremental; you do not have to have every data element perfect, but you do have to continually improve, and be particularly careful that the system and the data used do not make healthcare worse, or less safe than it was before the development was done.
7 Being mindful of information privacy concerns.
8 Minimising collector/recorder burden.
9 Using data development to reflect, not drive, practice.
10 Creating once, using often.
11 Having a governance process that includes expertise in data quality in information systems, but also includes representatives of data collectors and data users.

The data development processes outlined above includes the establishment and maintenance of data definitions, and is applicable to all healthcare areas where data are required. This includes the development of clinical data collections, including clinical-specialty-specific data collections. The processes outlined are relevant for local hospital data collections as well as state/territory or national data collections.

2.4 Security

When information is valued, we want to keep it safe. Safety involves safe storage (so that data are not lost), not letting those who shouldn't see the information gain access, and making sure that the information can be accessed when you want it. When using computers to store information, the situation is no different. Information can be lost when computer hardware fails. It can be damaged by the software used to produce and view it. People can access the data in the system and use it inappropriately, even if with the best of intentions.

To keep information in computer systems secure the data must be protected and so must the capacity to access that data through specific software techniques. Practical aspects of computer data security and retrieval are covered in Section 2.6.

2.4.1   Keeping stored information safe

Are there ever days when your car doesn't start? Can you think of any electrical device in your home or workplace that hasn't failed at some point in time? Computers are no different. And like many other elements of life, they will go wrong at the worst time.

Although computer storage appears stable and safe, it should be recognised that hard disks, memory sticks and CDs or DVDs should not be relied upon to last forever. This is both a factor of the media themselves – they are not guaranteed long-term storage devices – and of the fact that hardware change is very rapid. Ten years ago data were often stored on floppy disk drives; today, many computers no longer have the capacity to read these devices. Information stored on them is therefore no longer accessible and the data is, to all intents and purposes, lost.

For this reason a strategy for updating and managing your stored data should be considered for any valuable information. Periodic review, and copies or backup of all data, should be undertaken to keep it safe. More than one backup copy should be made, and they should ideally be stored on different sites (one at home and one at work, for example).

Backup options for personal use

To ensure data are not lost, store copies regularly using one or more of these options.

- Hard drive (C: drive)
  You could file a copy of the data files in an alternative location on your hard drive. Should your machine encounter difficulties, however, both the original file and the copy may become inaccessible or damaged. For this reason this option may be appropriate for the very short term, but it is not a sound strategy for protecting your work. If you have access to a second computer or a shared server, then backup copies may be placed there.
- CD or DVD
  This is probably the cheapest option, but again it cannot be expected to provide reliable long-term storage (although it can be useful in the short term, for example over the term of a project). If you wish to use CDs/DVDs for longer-term archiving, you will need to make at least two backup copies, stored on different sites, and set up a system to regularly review and re-copy the data onto new disks.
  Files stored to CD/DVD are generally not able to be modified unless they are copied back onto the hard drive.
- Memory stick
  These sticks can be plugged into a computer's USB port, and act like an extra hard drive for you to work on. They are fairly economical and a very versatile backup and alternative storage medium but, once again, cannot

be relied upon to last forever. For this reason it is important that you have more than one copy of your data, and backup regularly.

- External secure drive systems
  It is now possible to purchase hardware that not only can be plugged into computers that will hold large volumes of data (as much as your hard drive can hold), but that also comes with software that automatically ensures that your information is backed up regularly. These devices are decreasing in cost and increasing in capacity.

For organisations, the issue of backup and security is quite different. The technicalities of these requirements are not discussed here, as most organisations can be expected to have information technology departments responsible for these activities. However, it is relevant to understand that the same principles apply and that the technology can be used to provide more security and extensive backup provisions. Organisations in healthcare today often provide fully 'mirrored' systems where data stored is duplicated immediately at the time it is stored and software is run on more than one hardware device, enabling the system to keep operating 24 hours a day and being protected from individual device failures.

2.4.2 Privacy and access control

Health information is collected and used in manual systems for the purpose of direct patient care and with the implication that the patient has given consent for its usage. Beyond that, the use of health data is restricted in most countries by privacy legislation. Computers are excellent at presenting and retrieving health information. Although this has significant advantages in patient care, it also represents a threat to privacy. It is now easy to produce versions of health information that inadvertently breach the confidentiality of data. For example, a report may be produced that includes patient-identifying information and diagnostic information for clinical review. This document is useful for care and does not breach intended usage or trust; however, it must be destroyed effectively (shredded, or otherwise destroyed in a secure manner). Careless destruction of printed materials has caused privacy breaches in the past. The most common example is the discovery of paper-based patient information in rubbish dumps.

The general principles of confidentiality require that the information about an individual is protected. Confidentiality means that information you tell someone will remain confidential between you and that person unless there is a clear understanding that that information may be shared with others. In general, patients have the right to request that information not be shared, in which case the computer systems that manage that information must be able to comply with that request and ensure that only those authorised to see the information have access to it.

The issue of privacy is also an issue of trust. If the healthcare system is to function, patients must be able to trust that their data will be treated in a manner they find acceptable. The assumption that the patient is happy for any element of their medical history to be provided to any healthcare professional involved in their care is incorrect. There is an expectation among the healthcare-consumer community that relevant information will be provided to care providers, but this is not the same as providing open access to *everything*. Assumptions regarding the sensitivity of data should not be made either.

Example 2.7

Although information about sexually transmitted diseases and mental health are generally considered particularly sensitive, there are patients who, should they be admitted to hospital, would prefer that the history of their condition/s be made available as this is likely to lead to a faster and better health outcome. Healthcare consumers want to have *control* over the information made available. There are plenty of instances of patients restricting access to information that would not normally have been considered sensitive while being totally open about other parts of their history that some might think highly sensitive.

The issue of patients deciding not to reveal all of their health information is one that makes some healthcare professionals nervous. It is important to realise that this situation has always occurred; patients withhold information for many reasons. The only difference that arises as we move to computerised systems is the capacity of the computer system to identify that a patient has decided to restrict access to certain information. This capacity raises additional questions about the need to explain to patients the implication of not communicating their health information, although this is really no different to the pre-computer age. Patients do and have always needed to understand the importance of informing other healthcare providers of accurate medical history.

There are common requirements for privacy around the world. These requirements can be represented by looking at Australia's privacy principles, which are summarised below.[9] Other countries have laid out similar privacy principles, such as the UK's 1998 Data Protection Act.[10]

Principle 1 – Collection

Information must only be collected if it is required to support a specified function of the organisation, and that information must be collected only by lawful and fair means. In effect, this means that information should only be collected if it is to support patient care, or to meet a legal requirement such as reporting to authorised organisations (public health reporting).

The person from whom the information is obtained must reasonably understand:

- that the information is being collected
- the reason for that collection
- that they are able to access that information (they may request to see the information and have a person available to explain it to them if they desire)

- to whom the information is usually disclosed (other organisations or people) or who may have access to the information, e.g. clinical staff, administrative staff, government agencies for public health reporting, insurance agencies (access to the fact that a service was provided)
- where information is collected according to legal requirements, the law that requires such collection – for example, the collection and reporting of diagnoses for national public health data analysis, such as identification of the number of diabetes cases per year
- the consequences of not providing data – which is particularly relevant in clinical care. It is often difficult for patients to completely understand what is and is not relevant information in a given clinical situation. For example, a patient treated for painful knees may not realise that the treatment for arthritis is highly relevant to problems of heartburn and stomach complaints. It is important that clinical staff provide this information to the patient so that the patient understands that the knee condition may be relevant to the stomach condition (not an assumption most lay people would make).

Information should be collected from the actual person rather than third parties where this is possible; in clinical circumstances, this is not always able to be achieved. The cases where information is collected from others should occur with the patient's consent; or, where this is not possible, where it is in the best interest of the patient. There is an accepted convention that where information discovered would be detrimental to the patient if disclosed to them, this information can be restricted – but this action should be considered seriously and as a rare occurrence.

Principle 2 – Use and disclosure

Information collected for one purpose should not be disclosed or used for another (secondary) purpose unless:

- the secondary purpose is related to the primary purpose, and
- the individual would reasonably expect that this information would be shared, or
- where such access is the wish of the person concerned, such as release of information to the patient's family.

Example 2.8

Some information collected about a patient's admission to hospital, such as dates of admission, speciality and procedures/medications could reasonably be expected to be available to produce or support accounting and stores management functions within the organisation.

Information may be made available for the purpose of public health and safety and to support research, provided that this is done in a manner that protects the rights of the individual.

Providing access to information is also appropriate where:

- that access is provided in order to protect the individual to whom that information pertains
- there is reasonable suspicion of unlawful activity.

Principle 3 – Data quality

It is the responsibility of the organisation to take reasonable care that the information it 'collects, uses and discloses is accurate, complete and up to date'.

Principle 4 – Data security

The organisation must take steps to protect the security of the information in its care. When information is permanently de-identified (reference to individuals is removed from the data), that information is no longer needed for the purposes for which it was collected – the direct care of the patient – but is used and useful for long-term study of the health of our communities. The process of de-identification must ensure that all patients' information is no longer present, but also that it is not possible to infer or work out who a patient was by knowing, for example, their age, place of residence and disease.

Principle 5 – Openness

The organisation's policies for the management of personal information must be documented and freely available.

Principle 6 – Access and correction

A person must be given access to information held about them, except where such access would be detrimental to the patient's wellbeing. When such access is provided, the person is entitled to an explanation of the meaning of the information. In healthcare this often means that a person with clinical understanding must explain the terms and expressions used in the record in 'ordinary language'.

Principle 7 – Identifiers

Identifiers of an individual require the same access and disclosure protection as other pieces of information held about an individual, as access to the identifier may be used to gain access to other services or information about the individual.

Principle 8 – Anonymity

Individuals may elect to use pseudonyms to protect their identity when receiving services. This means that the person may use a different name to hide their identity. This is common practice when health professionals working in a specific area are treated, so that their privacy can be protected. It is also used for celebrities. Some pathology tests (such as HIV tests) are often sent using artificial or false names for the individual, as additional protection. The agency or clinician requesting or providing the service(s) is able to link the pseudonym back to the real data about the individual. Guidance on the principles of anonymity are provided in the international standard ISO TC215.[1]

Principle 9 – Trans-border data flows

Traditionally there have been legal and practical restrictions to the transfer of health information across state and national boundaries. The development of Electronic Health Records and more-integrated systems, such as the approach to healthcare service access in the European Union, require trans-border information flow. This process must be undertaken in a manner that protects the privacy of the individual's information and maintains the individual's expectations and instructions regarding disclosure.

Principle 10 – Sensitive information

An organisation should not collect sensitive information about an individual unless that information is needed to provide the service required by the individual, or to meet legal demands.

2.5 Ethical use of data

Data collected for one purpose – direct patient care – are used for other purposes that might not be so obvious to the patient. The data are used to support funding of healthcare; and are abstracted, summarised and sent to statistical units for monitoring the health of the nation. Most people expect that this occurs to some degree, but few understand how it occurs and how much data are collected.

Data collected in legally required reporting systems, such as those used to report the diseases and procedures performed in hospitals, provide a rich source of information. When these data are aggregated and produced as national statistics, they are not identifiable to an individual (de-identified data).

However, the extraction of data from any health data storage system, whether de-identified or not, should consider the privacy and ethical use of that data. Unfortunately, once data items are in a computer system, retrieving them can be so easy that there are many cases of inadvertent inappropriate access and use of patient information.

Clinical and health service research is governed by formal requirements for the ethical collection and handling of data, such as the National Statement on Ethical Conduct in Research Involving Humans.[11] Under these requirements, ethical collection, use and disclosure of health information will reflect patients' wishes regarding their information and meet legislative requirements for reporting of statistical information.

Ethical collection and use of data require either the use of public data that has been released through authorised agencies where de-identification has been undertaken and is guaranteed by these organisations, or data that has appropriate ethical clearance on its use. These include national data made available through the Internet, which can be considered public data.

When using identified or identifiable health data, it is important that the person to whom the data pertains has given permission for the use of that data, and that they are not pressured to participate nor put at risk by the data use. The International Standard on patient pseudonomisation provides guidelines on how to determine whether data is de-identified. This process is dependant upon the size of the population (the number of potential people in a data sample) and the variety in the data.

> ### Example 2.9
>
> A population of 100 people where there are 80 men and 20 women, divided into 10 age groups, may mean that in some age groups there is only one woman. If this is the case, the women would be considered identified.

It is appropriate to obtain ethics approval for the use of health data and to ensure that the methodology being used will represent the facts of the data correctly.

The requirement for ethics approval does not mean that data must be re-collected. The healthcare consumer assumes that existing data will be used when permission has been given, rather than expecting the patient to provide data again (duplicating data capture, and increasing the burden on the patient). The duplicate collection approach is common due to a misguided belief that keeping data in segregated collections will keep it safe. In today's systems, re-establishment of links to data are achievable for appropriate use and careful storage of data from existing systems and any additional data captured for the purpose of the research.

The responsibility to use health data ethically also requires that efforts be made to ensure the *accuracy* of data. Ethical use of extracted health data also require a disposal schedule for the data, where the storage, disposal and timetable for destruction are established ahead of the data collection.

Governments and research grant authorities around the world are increasingly requiring that information used in research activities be collected in a manner consistent with national health metadata definitions and code systems. This makes it more likely that the data can be used for longitudinal and comparative studies.

The length of time that data are kept in our systems is also changing. With the paper records of the past, the expense of filing space and data retrieval was significant and for this reason storage was limited, with formal disposal schedules for the destruction of records. In an electronic environment it may prove cheaper to keep records than to build archive systems to monitor and manage data. Certainly many healthcare consumers are seeking a lifelong record. The potential for significant research based upon these data is yet to be investigated.

EXERCISE 2.1

The questions below help you to consider how something that is quite simple to a person needs to be broken down into very small, precise, data components for a computer to process.

1   Using any clinical process, consider what the component data of the process are.
2   You have clinical data about a test result. How does a computer know that this result is outside the range of normal values?
3   You wish to investigate the treatment profiles of a group of patients with diabetes against their health outcomes. The data are in your computer system. Are there any privacy or ethical issues relevant to how this information can/should be used?
4   In what circumstances can you release information to a person other than the patient concerned?
5   Consider data you use regularly:
   ❏ Investigate metadata that defines the data and provides guidance on collection and use of that data.
   ❏ If you cannot find any published metadata for the type of data you collect or use regularly, describe the data component using the following headings:
      Data element name (field name)
      Definition
      Value domain (codes used)
      Guide for use (information for collectors or users of the data, including the purpose of collection).

2.6   Storage and retrieval

Any filing system that stores information must also make that information easy to find. If you cannot find it, there is little point in storing it in the first place! Computer systems have a standardised approach to the way files are managed.

2.6.1   Filename/s and properties

Each file in your computer has a name and a range of information stored about it (called *properties*). The filename has two components: the name section and the extension. The extension (or suffix) is the last three or four characters of the name – those characters that appear after the full stop.
   For example:

   letter to mary.doc

In this example the file extension is .doc (dot-doc). The file extension tells the system that runs your computer (the operating system) what program should be used to open the file. In the case of a .doc file, the program used is Microsoft Word. Examples of file extensions are shown in Table 2.1.

Table 2.1 Some common file extensions

File extension	Software associated with the suffix
csv	comma-separated variables *or* comma-separated values (such files may be opened by many programs, but often will make little sense unless opened by spreadsheet software)
doc	Microsoft Word document
docx	Microsoft Word 2007 (or 2008 for Mac) document
jpg	picture format often used on the Internet
mdb	Microsoft Access database
pdf	portable document format; this format is used to transfer information in a manner that cannot easily be altered and is therefore preferred as a legal record of communication
pps	Microsoft PowerPoint slide show
ppt	Microsoft PowerPoint presentation
pptx	Microsoft PowerPoint 2007 (or 2008 for Mac) presentation
rtf	rich text format (developed for cross-platform document exchange; most word-processors can read and alter .rtf files)
txt	plain text format (a file containing text with very little formatting, which can be opened by a wide range of programs)
xls	Microsoft Excel spreadsheet
xlsx	Microsoft Excel 2007 (or 2008 for Mac) spreadsheet
zip	files compressed by zip compression software

You can change a file extension by renaming a file. This process doesn't change the content of the file – what changes is the ability to automatically identify the software used to open that file.

Example 2.10

If you change the name of the file *letter to mary.doc* to *letter to mary.xxx*, the computer will no longer display the Word icon next to the file name.

If you then double-click on the new filename, you will be asked what software to use. If you have Word running and open *letter to mary.xxx* from within Word, the document will open without a problem.

If you then change the name back to the original *letter to mary.doc* the file would again display the Word icon, and automatically open using Word software were to you double-click on it.

How do you know the file suffix if you can't see it?

Your computer may have been originally set up without showing file extensions; this is quite common. To view your files go to **Start ➤ My Documents** (Fig 2.3).

Figure 2.3
Filenames
without file
extensions

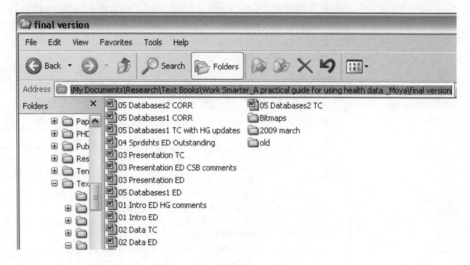

To see the file extensions you must change the folder options for Windows. To do this:

1 Go to **Tools ➤ Folder Options**. Figure 2.4 shows the Folder Options dialog box.
2 Go to the **View** tab (Fig 2.5).

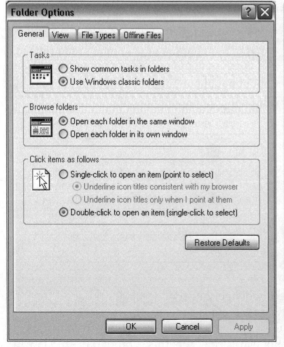

Figure 2.4 Folder Options dialog box

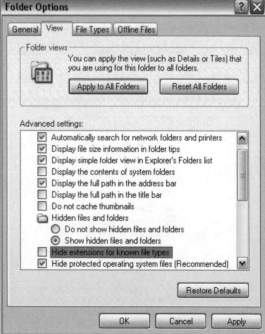

Figure 2.5 Folder Options – View tab

This area allows you to change what you are shown in the display of your files. To see file extensions, left-click on the box to the left of 'Hide extensions for known file types' to remove the tick mark. (It is the last of the items shown in Figure 2.5). Left-click **Apply to All Folders** then **OK**, and the display will change. It will now look like the one shown in Figure 2.6.

Figure 2.6
Folder display
with extensions

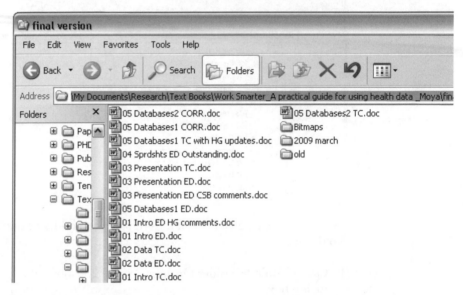

You can also change what information is provided about each file. Look at Figure 2.7 – here you can also see file size, the date the file was last modified, and the file type (which determines which program will open that file).

Figure 2.7 Display of file details

To see these details, you need to change the view type by clicking on the **Views** icon (Fig 2.8). The view type **Details** provides the more extensive view, and is particularly useful for version control where knowing the date the file was last saved is key. You can also access this submenu from **View** in the top menu.

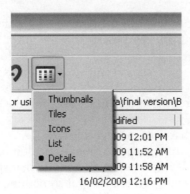

Figure 2.8 View types

2.6.2 Filing systems

When you file paper documents, you have many options, for example: you can pile them on the floor, put them in a drawer, sort them into folders that are filed alphabetically with a new version each year so that you can throw out the old versions. You might need to make sure that others in your home or organisation can access your stored paper when you are away or ill. Computer filing is no different.

A filing system requires a system of classification that groups common things together, and a method of identifying what you have filed. The structure you use for filing is made up of folders. You can create folders in any area of your computer system, but it is recommended that you keep your information in the 'My Documents' area, or your organisation's specified filing area (which might be a specific drive on the machine). Where information is stored on a shared computer device, or server, the file structure should be agreed and understood by all. Where it is on your own computer the issue of standardisation is less important, but you still need to be consistent in your approach to filing structure and the naming of files.

Folder structure
The folder structure should have the following features:

* Be mutually exclusive – there should only be one logical place where you put things on any given topic.
  A good example for articles is that they could be filed by author (first author if there is more than one). A less-clear example would be filing articles by topic; many articles cover more than one topic.
* Be given a meaningful title that will assist you in finding the document. For example, filing meeting notes by date is meaningful. However, if you record the date as '5 May 08', the notes will not sort by the date of the meeting, but alphabetically by title:
  7 Aug 08
  5 May 08
  9 Sep 08.

If you name the meeting notes with the date as numbers in reverse order, they will sort correctly for your purposes:

2008_05_05
2008_08_07
2008_09_09

This also allows you to archive folders into years, for older information.

- Have a folder structure that is of manageable size.
  The larger the folder structure gets, the more difficult it is to find the components you seek. It is important to remember that storage is of no value if you can't remember where you put something. The folder structure should be sufficiently wide (the number of folders at any given level) to represent the broad categories of information you need to access without requiring more than five levels of depth (folders within folders). In this way, access to any given file won't take too long (require too many clicks). An example is shown in Figure 2.9.

Figure 2.9 My Documents folder structure

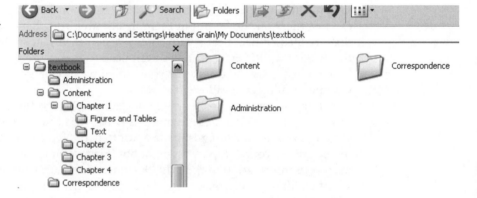

Naming files

Once you have established a folder structure, you must also consider the actual naming conventions for your files. This is particularly important where you collect or create multiple versions of a document as you add to and change it – it should always be clear which is the latest version (Fig 2.10).
Useful techniques include:

- descriptive filenames
- using numerals in filenames and folder names to keep them in chronological order
- including your initials and/or the date in a filename.

For example, if someone sends you a file to be amended, first save a copy with your initials (and perhaps date) included in the name. Modify *this* file and return it. Because the filename is different, the other person will be able to save it to the appropriate folder without the danger of overwriting the original file. The integrity of the original file is thus maintained, and it is easy to compare the two to see the changes.

Figure 2.10
Numbering files and folders to maintain order

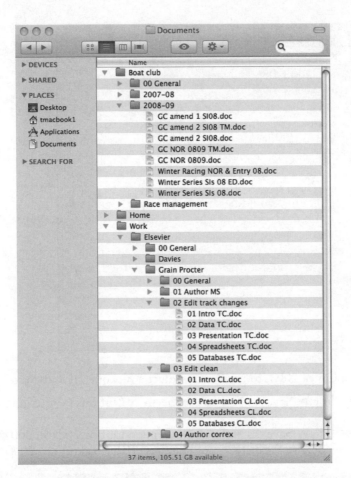

2.6.3 Locks and passwords

Where you have a document that you don't want others to change, you can protect it with a password. This means that others cannot open and/or modify the document unless you have given them the document password.

In general, it is wise not to use your normal system password on documents you intend to share. Allocation and choice of passwords is always a difficulty, but there are some basic rules. Strong passwords mix number and characters but are still easy for you to remember. For example, P110t is like 'pilot' but using numbers to replace the letters. This is less strong if everyone knows you are a mad keen pilot – the principle is sound but don't choose a word or context that people associate with you or with the job you do. An example of a poor password is 'adm1t' for the admissions office. Also, longer passwords are stronger; try to use at least eight characters.

In Office 2007, to password-protect a file, open it and go to:

• **Office Button ➤ Save As ➤ Options ➤ General Options** (Word 2007, PowerPoint 2007, Excel 2007)
• **Database Tools ➤ Encrypt with Password** (Access 2007).

Figure 2.11
General security
options in Word
2007

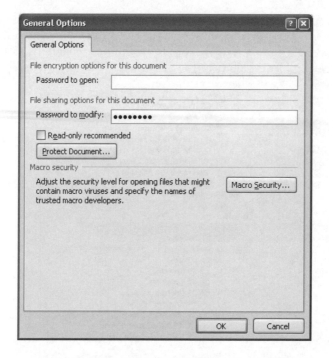

In Office 2003, to password-protect a file, open it and go to:

- **File ➤ Save As ➤ Tools ➤ Security Options** (Word 2003, PowerPoint 2003)
- **File ➤ Save As ➤ Tools ➤ General Options** (Excel 2003)
- **Tools ➤ Security ➤ Set Database Password** (Word 2003, Access 2003).

Figure 2.12
Security options
in Word 2003

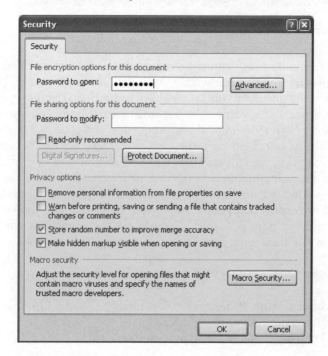

Quick hint

Note that protection of databases works differently to other programs; it is best to search for 'password' in Access Help to see all the different options and how to apply them.

You can generally encrypt the file so that a password is required to open it, and a different password to modify it. You can use these options separately, or apply both together. The password will show as a series of black dots when you enter it.

Office 2007 also offers more secure encryption, by going to:

* **Office Button ➤ Prepare ➤ Encrypt Document** (Fig 2.13).

Figure 2.13
Encrypting a 2007 document

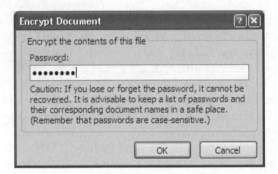

The **Prepare** submenu (available for Word 2007, PowerPoint 2007 and Excel 2007) has a number of different options you may want to set before you distribute a document (Fig 2.14).

Figure 2.14
Prepare submenu in Office 2007

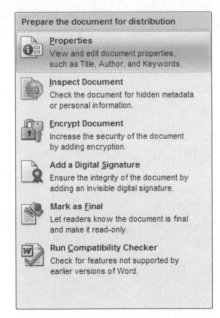

References

1. ISO TC 215, Technical Committee on Health Information Technology, *17115 Health Informatics: Vocabulary of Terminological Systems*. Geneva: ISO; 2007.
2. ISO TC 215, Technical Committee on Health Information Technology, *25237 Health Informatics: Pseudonomysation*. Geneva: ISO, 2008.
3. Standards Australia, *AS5021 The Language of Health Concept Representation*. Sydney: Standards Australia IT14, 2005.
4. Olson J, *Data Quality: the accuracy dimension*, 5th edn. Morgan Kaufmann, 2003.
5. National Centre for Classification in Health, ed, *The International Statistical Classification of Diseases and Related Health Problems, Tenth Revision, Australian Modification (ICD-10-AM)*, 5th edn. Sydney: NCCH, 2006.
6. Australian Institute of Health and Welfare, *Metadata Online Registry (METeOR)*. Canberra: AIHW, 2005. Available from: http://meteor.aihw.gov.au/content/index.phtml/itemId/181162 [7 June 2009].
7. ISO/IEC 11179, *standard for Information Technology, Metadata Registries*. Available from: http://metadata-stds.org/11179/index.html [12 June 2009].
8. International Organization for Standardization. www.iso.org.
9. The Privacy Amendment (Private Sector) Act 2000. Available from www.privacy.gov.au/publications/npps01.html [9 June 2009].
10. Data Protection Act 1998. HMSO: London. Available from: http://www.opsi.gov.uk/Acts/Acts1998/ukpga_19980029_en_1 [21 May 2009].
11. National Health and Medical Research Council, Australian Research Council and Australian Vice-Chancellors' Committee, *National Statement of Ethical Conduct in Human Research*. Canberra: Australian Government, 2007.

3   Presentation and sharing

Learning objectives

When this chapter is completed you will:
- have an understanding of some places and ways you can share your information
- know how to use Word to present information
- be able to create a simple PowerPoint presentation
- know of, and have tried, some ways of presenting information on the Internet
- know what impacts the method of sharing can have on confidentiality
- know how to create a PDF file.

One of the mistakes many people make when planning how to present their information is to start by thinking about the *information*. Actually, the best place to start is with the *target audience*. Who your audience is – and how you will interact with that audience – will affect how you present your information.

Once you know the audience for your information, you can start thinking about how to structure it to help your audience understand what it is that you have to say.

- If you have to do a 'live' presentation to a group of people, a presentation package such as PowerPoint will help you.
- If you won't be able to meet your audience face to face but know who they are, then some type of written format that can be sent via email or as hard (printed) copy will be necessary. This could be as simple as using a word processing package (although please also note the section on PDF files).
- If you know the *type* of people who you want to see your information but don't actually know the individuals' names or contact information, then a web-based format is likely to be the most effective.

Table 3.1 shows some examples of information for different audiences and gives suggestions for methods of presentation.

Table 3.1 Suggested formats for communicating to different audiences

You are a:	Your information is:	Your audience is:	Suggested format:
Student	An assessed presentation	Lecturers	Presentation package
Health administrator	Clinic attendance report for the previous month	Manager	Word-processed document
Health service manager	Proposal to open a new walk-in clinic service	Board/Directors	Structured, word-processed report. If presenting to a board meeting, also a presentation package
Nurse	Results of a study about patient user groups	Patients and healthcare professionals	Internet

As mentioned in the Introduction, we will be giving detailed instructions for the Microsoft applications Word 2007 and Word 2003.

3.1 Using Word effectively

Learning objectives

When this section is completed you will be able to:

- use the features of Word
- choose appropriate features of Word to present information effectively
- understand the relationship of Word to other software packages, and be able to use this functionality to support presentation of information.

Microsoft Word is one of the most common methods of presenting information. There is a need to be able to use Word effectively to present information in the most effective and appropriate manner. There are some general tools that can be used within Word to assist in presentation of data. These are described below with examples for you to try.

3.1.1 Page setup and printing options

The layout of data in a Word document can be presented in different ways according to the way the page is set up. **Page Setup** governs the size and orientation of the page, as well as the margins, shading and colours, borders and paragraphs (any text that finishes with an Enter key), and many other elements. It is always a good idea to check your page setup before you start working on a document (although of course you may always change things later).

*   In Word 2007, go to the **Page Layout** ribbon and click on the small arrow to the right of **Page Setup**.

*   In Word 2003, go to **File ➤ Page Setup**.

A dialogue box similar to Figure 3.1 will be displayed.

Figure 3.1 Page Setup dialog box – **Margins** tab

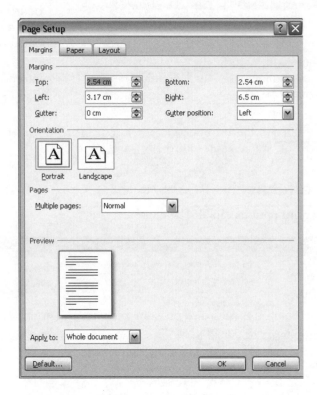

Margins tab

Here the **margins** can be made smaller or larger. Be careful not to make them too small – if the print area goes outside the paper or printer's capacity, a warning message will be given when you try to print the document.

Orientation changes the direction of printing on the paper.

When you modify the page setup you can apply the change to the **whole document** (as in Figure 3.1), or can choose to modify the setup of sections or pages of the document, or to a specific selected area of the text.

Paper tab

The **Paper** tab is displayed in Figure 3.2. This allows the user to select the size of the paper to be used, and to indicate if the first page of the document is to be printed from a different printer tray (for example, headed notepaper) than the other pages. Word normally comes set up with the paper size Letter (or US Letter), and if you are printing on A4 it is best to choose this size to avoid parts of your document being cut off when printing.

Figure 3.2 Page Setup – **Paper** tab

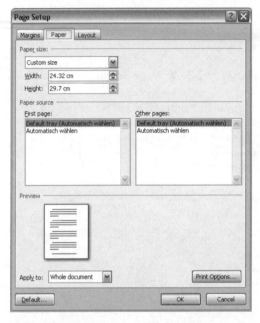

Special print options can also be chosen.

Figure 3.3 Print options in Word 2007

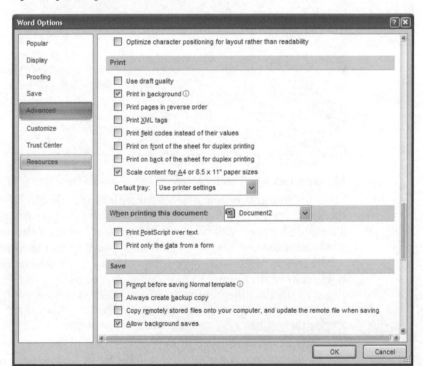

- In Word 2007, clicking on the **Print Options** button will bring up the **Word Options** dialog box. Select **Advanced** and scroll down to find the **Print** options (Fig 3.3).
- In Word 2003, simply click on the **Print Options** button to bring up a dialogue box (Fig 3.4).

Figure 3.4 Print options in Word 2003

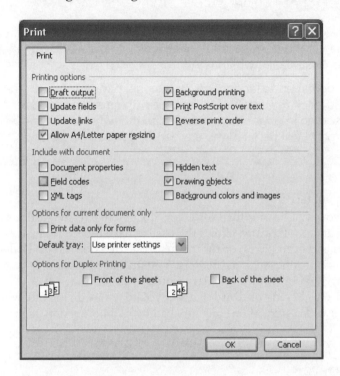

Print options can be used to manage the quality and process of printing the document you are working on. The ability to **reverse the print order** is particularly useful for large documents if you normally have to re-sort your pages after they are printed. You can also control whether the document prints any pictures or drawing objects within it.

Quick hint

Word allows you to change the settings for a particular document, or for all documents to personalise your copy of the program. Be cautious with permanent personalisations if you are working on a shared machine.

In Word 2007, these settings are accessed through the Word Options screen, for example the Popular, Display, Proofing and Save tabs.

In Word 2003, they are found under the Tools item in the menu bar; most are in a dialog box accessed through the path Tools ➤ Options, and are grouped into appropriate tabs like View, Spelling and Grammar, Save.

EXERCISE 3.1

Open the sample document *Exercise 3-1.doc* provided on the CD and save it to an appropriate location on your computer.

1   Change the size of the paper. The sample document provided is in Letter size, commonly used in the USA but not consistent with the standard letter size used in Europe and Australasia, which is A4.

2   Change the orientation to landscape for a single paragraph in the sample document, and back to portrait. Observe how the margins and the look of the page on the screen change. You should note that when changes like this are made, a new page will begin at the start and end of the orientation change.

Layout tab

Layout can be modified for whole documents, or for sections of the document. This area allows the user to have different headers and footers for odd and even pages, or for the first page of a document. It also controls the position of headers and footers. You may need to adjust these to make sure they print on your particular printer.

Left-clicking on **Borders** takes you to a new dialog box where you can set up a wide range of options for shading and borders on pages and paragraphs.

Figure 3.5 Page Setup – **Layout** tab

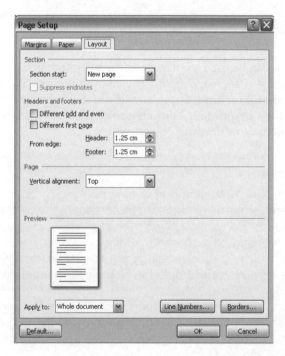

'Default' button

Note the **Default** button that shows on all three tabs of Page Setup. This is very useful if you plan to use the same basic page setup for most of your documents. After you have set up your document and checked it by doing a test print, left-click the **Default** button – from now on, all your Word documents will open with your chosen setup. Of course, you can still change page setup for individual documents if you need something different.

Print preview

Page details can also be modified through the **Print Preview** option. To see a print preview:

- in Word 2007, go to **Office Button** ➤ **Print** ➤ **Print Preview**
- in Word 2003, go to **File** ➤ **Print Preview**, or left-click on the Print Preview icon on the icon bar (Fig 3.6).

Figure 3.6 Print Preview icon

Print Preview
Preview and make changes to pages before printing.

The result is shown in Figure 3.7.

Print Preview allows the user to change the margins of the document interactively. Margins can be changed by left-clicking and holding on the border inside the ruler, and dragging the margin to a new location.

Figure 3.7 Print Preview margin controls

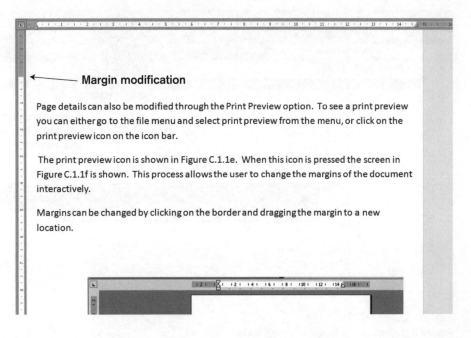

3.1.2   Using columns

Information is often easier to read and can have a more interesting layout when presented in 'newspaper' style with multiple columns. To create columns, select the text you want to appear in columns, then:

- in Word 2007, go to **Page Layout ➤ Columns** (Fig 3.8)
- in Word 2003, left-click the column icon (Fig 3.9).

Figure 3.8
Column options
in Word 2007

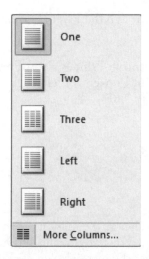

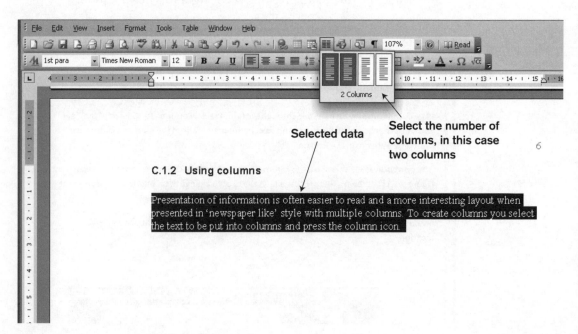

Figure 3.9 Creating columns in Word 2003

The result of this process is shown in Figure 3.10.

Presentation

Presentation of information is often easier to read and more interesting when presented in 'newspaper like' style with multiple columns. To create columns you select the text to be put into columns and press the column icon

Figure 3.10 Columns created

To get columns to balance nicely, sometimes you want to break a column over to the next column (or page). Place your cursor at the beginning of the text that you want to move into a new column, then:

- in Word 2007, go to **Page Layout ➤ Breaks**
- in Word 2003, go to **Insert ➤ Break**

and chose the type of break you want.

3.1.3 Inserting pictures and/or drawings

Pictures, charts and other images can be inserted into Word documents. One way this can be done is to simply copy and paste into the document. When this simple approach is taken the image is structured as if it is text. It can be positioned against the left or right border or centred, and it may appear cut off at the top (this happens when you have a fixed line spacing for your paragraphs).

A more flexible way is to format the layout of the pasted picture as 'square' – then you will be able to move it around, and the text will wrap around the picture. To do this, **select** the picture, **right-click** and choose **Format Picture**. Choose **Square** and click on **OK**. You can now move the picture around using click-and-drag. The Format Picture dialog box can also be used to resize or crop the image, add a line outside it, etc.

Figure 3.11
Options for formatting a picture

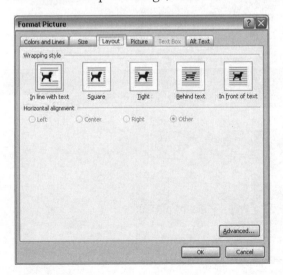

Another option is to inserted the image into a 'drawing' or text box. An advantage of this is that it allows you to add a caption and keep the two elements together when you move them. The use of text boxes is discussed below.

Drawings and shapes

To be able to use drawing facilities, you need to have the Drawing toolbar active.

- In Word 2007, the Drawing toolbar will display once you have inserted a line, shape, or new drawing canvas. Go to **Insert ➤ Shapes**. Here, click on the line or shape you want to use (Fig 3.12) and move to your page to start drawing – the Drawing Tools toolbar will appear at the top of your Word window. Alternatively, you can choose **New Drawing Canvas** at the bottom of the list in **Shapes**, and again the Drawing Tools toolbar will appear.
- In Word 2003, go to **View ➤ Toolbars** and select the **Drawing** toolbar (ensure there is a tick in the box next to 'Drawing').The screen will show the Drawing toolbar, often at the foot of your Word window, as shown in Figure 3.13. Now, left-click on the line or shape you want and start drawing.

Figure 3.12
Shape options in Word 2007

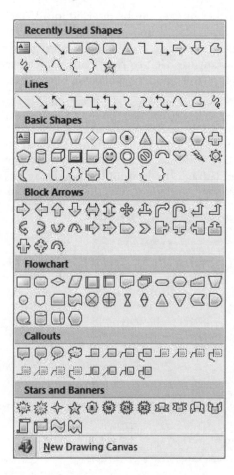

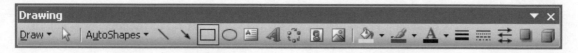

Figure 3.13 Drawing toolbar in Word 2003

Alternative drawing objects can be used (Fig 3.14).

Figure 3.14
Drawing object
options (Word
2003)

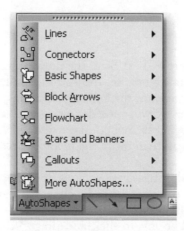

There are also options that manage the relative position of drawing objects: they can be sent behind or in front of text, or of other objects; they can be rotated or grouped together (where multiple objects are joined so that they can be manipulated as if they were one item). These options can be accessed by clicking on the object you want to manipulate, then:

• in Word 2007, through the 'Arrange' section of the Drawing Tools toolbar
• in Work 2003 in the Drawing toolbar, go to **Draw ➤ Order** and choose the correct option.

Image and text boxes

When images or special text are included in a document, they can be inserted into a text box that you can move around freely into the desired position on the page. Both text and images can be inserted into the same box.

A disadvantage is that the text in text boxes doesn't get saved if the document is saved to a different format, e.g. if it is converted to a plain text file before being used in a different program. If your document is likely to be treated in this way, an alternative option is to use a single-celled table and insert the picture and caption into that. This is not as flexible to move around, but it will save rekeying 'lost' text (tables are discussed later).

To insert into a Word document an image or a block of text that you can move around freely, use the Text Box tool. This inserts a box that can be positioned in any place within the document (the resulting box can be clicked and dragged; its size changed; its colour and outlines modified; and so on).

- In Word 2007, go to **Insert ➤ Text Box ➤ Simple Text Box**. The following box will appear (Fig 3.15). To get rid of the text, left-click in the middle of the paragraph and hit **Backspace**.

Figure 3.15 Text Box in Word 2007

[Type a quote from the document or the summary of an interesting point. You can position the text box anywhere in the document. Use the Text Box Tools tab to change the formatting of the pull quote text box.]

- In Word 2003, go to **Insert ➤ Text Box**. The mouse image (cursor) changes to a + sign. To draw a box, set the + in the top left corner position of about where you want the box, and left-click, hold and drag to the bottom right corner. (If you get a drawing canvas that you can't get rid off, try click-and-dragging from a point outside the drawing canvas – it should disappear. You can then move the box to where you want it.)

When the text box is selected, it has small squares or circles in each corner and in the middle of each of the edge lines. To **change the size of the box** put your cursor over any of these small shapes. When your cursor changes to a **two-headed arrow** you will be able to click-and-drag to change the size or shape of the box.

To **move** the whole box, place your cursor on one of the edge lines but away from any of the small shapes. Your cursor will change to a **four-headed arrow**. Left-click, hold and drag the whole box to where you want it.

To **format** the box (for example to remove the line around the outside or add a fill colour), select the box and right-click. Be careful to select the actual box rather than any text inside it. Choose **Format Text Box** from the dialog box that appears.

Figure 3.16 Text Box tool in Word 2003, with added image and text

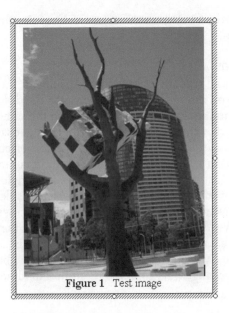

Figure 1   Test image

To **add text**, simply click inside the box and type. To **add an image of your own** into the box, click inside the box then go to:

- **Insert ➤ Picture** (Word 2007)
- **Insert ➤ Picture ➤ From File** (Word 2003)

and choose your image. It will appear inside the box (Fig 3.16).

Captions can be put into the text box by the image, or by pictures simply inserted into documents. These can be automatically numbered and will be able to have an automatic Table of Figures created by Word. To add a caption, put your cursor on the image and move the cursor one space to the right, then press the return key to put your cursor on a new line underneath the image.

- In Word 2007, go to **References ➤ Insert Caption.**
- In Word 2003, go to **Insert ➤ Reference ➤ Caption.**

This will produce the dialog box shown in Figure 3.17.

A similar process can be used to add captions to tables, if you want them to be automatically numbered.

Figure 3.17
Automated
captions

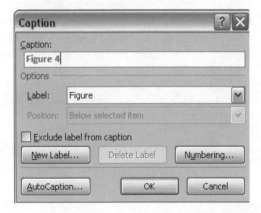

EXERCISE 3.1 CONTINUED

3 In the sample document *Exercise 3-1.doc*, select a block of text and make it double-column. Experiment with different column layouts to get an attractive and readable layout, leaving the preface single-column and inserting a page break before the section heading.

4 Place the sample picture supplied (or use one of your own) in the sample document, formatting it as 'square' layout. Resize it to a single column width and place it on the right-hand side in an appropriate position.

5 Insert a text box at the end of the sample document. Add a picture and caption to the text box. Size the image and caption appropriately, and centre it below the end of the text.

3.1.4   Headings (titles)

Word offers features to help format the style of your document consistently, and is particularly useful for titles within the document.

Word 2007 styles

Word 2007 comes with a range of different styles from which you can choose, visible in the **Home** ribbon (Fig 3.18). The **Change Styles** button allows you to choose from a range of inbuilt style sets. You can preview how the styles will look in your document by positioning your cursor in the middle of a paragraph and hovering over a style in the ribbon.

It is often helpful to open the **Styles** panel by clicking on the small blue arrow at the bottom right of the Styles section of the ribbon, and then selecting **Show Preview**. This shows you a fuller range of styles, and you can also add new styles by clicking on the **New Style** button. To **modify** a style, hover over it in the Styles panel and left-click the down-arrow that appears.

Figure 3.18
Style sets in
Word 2007

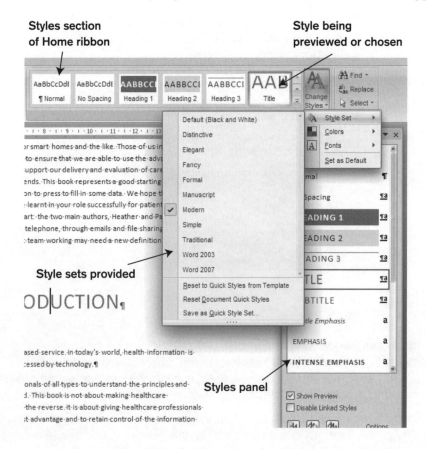

**Styles section
of Home ribbon**

**Style being
previewed or chosen**

Style sets provided

Styles panel

Word 2003

In Word 2003, go to **Format ➤ Styles and Formatting** to bring up the **Styles and Formatting** panel (Fig 3.19). Choose to show 'Available Styles' if this is not already selected, as otherwise the list of styles will be overly long. You can also apply styles from the Formatting toolbar by clicking on the down-arrow to the right of the style box and selecting the required style.

To **modify** a style, hover over it in the Styles panel and left-click the down-arrow that appears. Add a new style with the **New Style** button.

Figure 3.19
Styles and Formatting panel in Word 2003, showing the basic styles provided

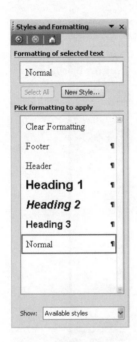

Applying styles

To apply styles, place your cursor in the middle of the paragraph you want to style and click on the style you want. To style two (or more) consecutive paragraphs at once, click in the middle of a paragraph and drag your cursor down to the middle of the next paragraph, then choose your style.

Document templates

You can save a modified set of styles as a document template which you can then attach to another document. This is particularly useful if you want a uniform look to be applied to a range of documents, for example sections of a long report.

To save a document template:

- in Word 2007, go to **Office Button ➤ Save As ➤ Word Template**
- in Word 2003, go to **File ➤ Save As** and choose **Document Template (*.dot)** in the **Save as type** area.

To attach a document template:

- in Word 2007, go to **Office Button ➤ Word Options ➤ Add-ins**, select 'Templates' in the **Manage** list, and click on **Go**
- in Word 2003, go to **Tools ➤ Templates and Add-Ins**.

Left-click on **Attach** and choose your template. Choose to automatically update document styles, and click on **OK**.

Figure 3.20
Attaching a document template

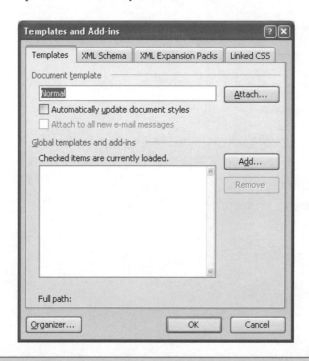

EXERCISE 3.1 CONTINUED

6   In the sample document *Exercise 3-1.doc*, apply the supplied 'Title' style to the preface heading and the section heading. Modify the heading to bold and centre it. Apply other heading styles as appropriate.

7   Create a new style 'Preface text', making it Arial 10pt and indented left and right by 1.5 cm. Apply the style to the preface main text.

8   (Self-study) Save the document under a new name and experiment with styles to produce other attractive and clear presentations. Save these as templates if you wish.

3.1.5 Tables

Tables are common tools used to present data. A useful feature is that you can simply copy a table in a Word document and paste it into a spreadsheet – and the cell structure will be retained. A cell is one 'square' of the table.

Inserting tables in Word 2007

To add a table, go to the **Insert** ribbon and left-click the **Tables** button. You will be shown a grid from which you can decide the number of rows and columns you need in the table.

Figure 3.21
Inserting a table in Word 2007

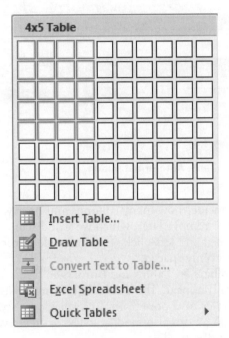

You need to briefly consider how many columns and rows you will need – you can always add or remove later, which we will discuss a little later. Highlight what you need and left-click.

The table will automatically be created with columns evenly spaced, and the **Design** section of the Table Tools ribbon will be shown (Fig 3.22). Here you choose from a variety of styles or create your own. Hover over a style in the ribbon to preview it; click to apply.

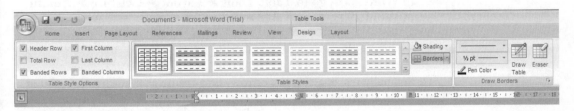

Figure 3.22 Design section of Table Tools ribbon

Inserting tables in Word 2003

Click on the **Table** icon in the menu bar. You will be shown a grid from which you can decide the number of rows and columns you need in the table.

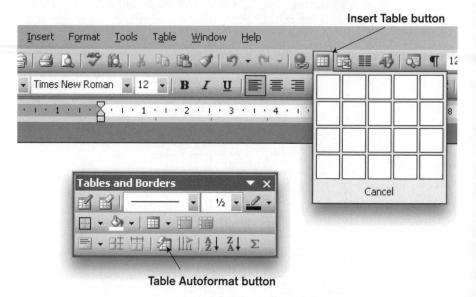

Insert Table button

Table Autoformat button

You need to briefly consider how many columns and rows you will need – you can always add or remove later, which we will discuss a little later. Highlight what you need and left-click. The table will automatically be created with columns evenly spaced.

Go to **View ➤ Toolbars ➤ Tables and Borders** to bring up the toolbar if it does not automatically appear. The **Table Autoformat** button (Fig 3.23) gives you a range of styles to choose from. Left-click on a style to preview it; click on **Apply** to use. You can also modify styles, or create your own using the line and fill tools in the toolbar.

Managing tables

To add data to your table, left-click in a cell and type. You can use the **Autofit** option to find the best column size to fit the data you have included in the table, or set the column and row sizes manually.

- To use Autofit, left-click somewhere inside your table. Then:
  - in Word 2007, go to **Table Tools ➤ Layout ➤ Cell Size ➤ Autofit**
  - in Word 2003, go to **Table ➤ AutoFit**

and choose from the options available (Fig 3.24).

- To manually resize a column or row, first ensure that automatic resizing of a table is turned off. Then hover over a column (or row) line until the cursor changes to a pair of short lines with outward-pointing arrows. Click-and-drag to resize.

Figure 3.24
AutoFit options

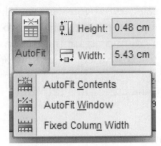

Table **headings** can be established by merging cells across a row, or up or down a table for side headings. To merge cells, click-and-drag to select the cells to be joined and right-click to bring up a dialog box (Fig 3.25). Select Merge Cells; the result is shown in Figure 3.26. Note all the other table management options you can access with a right-click.

Figure 3.25
Merging cells

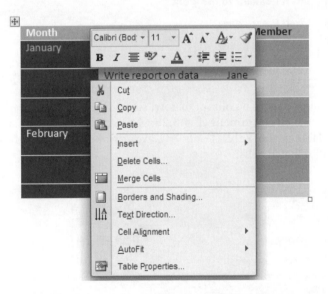

Figure 3.26
Result of merging
cells

Month	Action Required	Staff Member
January	Build requirements document	Mary
	Write report on data protection	Jane
	Prepare project documentation	Alex
February	Prepare research material	Jane
	Demonstrate new processes	Mary

To **delete** a row or column, first select what you wish to delete. For a row, hover over the far left of the row until the cursor changes to an arrow. For a column, hover over the top of the column; again the cursor will change to an arrow. Left-click to select the entire row or column. Now press the **Delete** key.

To **add** a row or column, place the cursor in a cell either side of the area you want to add. Then:

- for Word 2007, right-click and select **Insert**
- for Word 2003, go to **Table ➤ Insert**.

Figure 3.27 shows the options you are given.

Figure 3.27
Inserting a
column or row

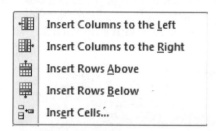

To **align** data in a column or row, select the area concerned, right-click and choose **Cell Alignment** (Fig 3.28). In Word 2007 these same buttons are available in the **Table Tools ➤ Layout** ribbon. The modifications will apply to all selected cells.

Figure 3.28 Cell
alignment options

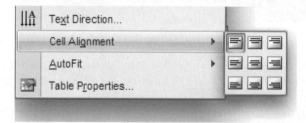

A useful way of aligning numerals in columns is to use a decimal tab. First make sure that the rulers are visible in your document. If they are not:

- for Word 2007, go to the **View** ribbon, and in **Show/Hide** select **Ruler**
- for Word 2003, go to **View ➤ Ruler**.

Where the rulers meet in the top left-hand corner, there is a little tab mark in a square. Left-click this several times until the decimal tab mark is showing (Fig 3.29). Now highlight the cells in one column you want to decimal-align. Move your cursor up to the top ruler, and click in the middle of the ruler relating to that column. The tab mark will appear on the ruler and your numerals will be decimal-aligned.

Figure 3.29
Using a decimal
tab to align
numerals

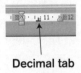

Decimal tab

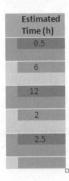

3.1.6 Merging data from another source

Word provides the option of taking data from a spreadsheet or database and using automated processes to produce documents. An example is a standard letter where each individual's details are taken from a database and inserted into fields in a Word document. This produces multiple individualised letters from one document.

EXERCISE 3.2

The worked example in this exercise uses the database file *patients.mdb* provided on the CD. You can either access the file directly on the CD or copy it to your computer.

We are going to use this to create a letter to be given to patients when they arrive at an organisation. The letter is to include each individual's record number and name.

Figure 3.30 shows what information we want to include in the standard letter.

Figure 3.30
Information to be shown in standard letter (merging exercise)

> Date
>
> 'Record Number'
>
> 'Name'
>
>
> Dear 'Given Name'
>
>
> Thank you for attending the hospital today. We are training new staff today and apologise for any delays you might experience. We will do our best to look after you as quickly as possible.

Open a new, blank Word document. Now we need to open the Mail Merge Wizard:

- in Word 2007, go to **Mailings ➤ Start Mail Merge ➤ Step by Step Mail Merge Wizard**
- in Word 2003, go to **Tools ➤ Letters and Mailings ➤ Mail Merge**.

To the right of your Word window, the Mail Merge Wizard will open; we will now work through it.

Figure 3.31
Menu for mail merging (Word 2007)

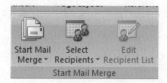

Step 1
Choose **Letters,** then (at the bottom of the panel) left-click on **Next: Starting document**.

Figure 3.32 Mail Merge document type selection

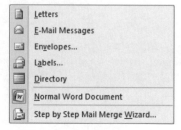

Step 2

Select **Use the current document,** as you will create the document in the blank Word document currently open. Go to **Next: Select recipients**.

Step 3

Choose **Use an existing list** and then **Browse** to find and choose the *patients. mdb* file. You will then be asked to choose the table that contains the data required (Fig 3.33).

Figure 3.33
Select the table that contains the data needed in the merge process

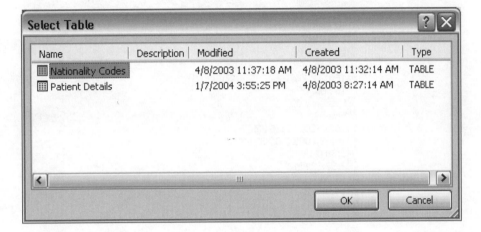

Select the **Patient Details** table. Now you will see a display of the content of the table and its structure. You will need to indicate which entries are to be included in the merge (Fig 3.34). In this example we are to include all recipients, so choose **Select All** and go to **Next: Write your letter**.

Figure 3.34 Mail Merge data components in the Patient Details table

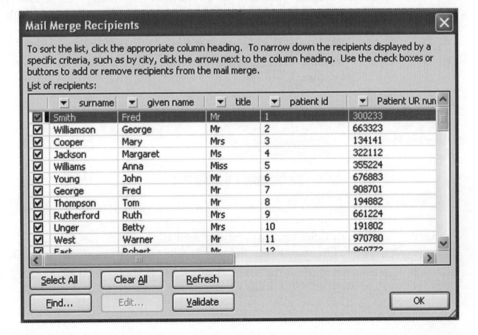

Step 4

When writing the letter, the first step is to add the date. To do this go to **Insert ➤ Date and Time**. This will allow you to insert a date automatically of the format you choose (Fig 3.35).

Figure 3.35 Date and Time formats

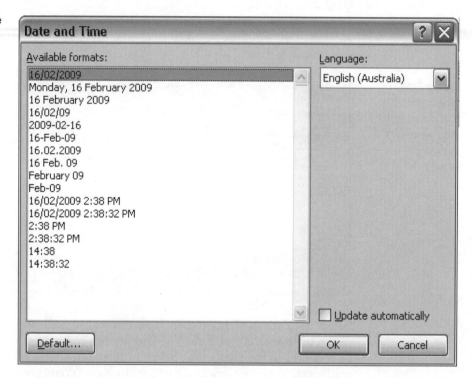

To add the patient's record number and name, choose the **More items** option in the right-hand Mail Merge panel – all of the database fields in the Patient Details database will be offered. Select the record number and left-click **Insert**; then insert the title, given name and surname in the same way. Close the dialog box. As items are selected they will appear on the letter as in Figure 3.36.

Figure 3.36 Inserting field entries in a Mail Merge

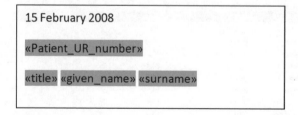

Continue until you have placed all the fields you want.

To separate the fields out, select each individual entry, and enter a space or a return, as needed. Type in the text of the letter; your document should now look like Figure 3.37.

Figure 3.37
Completed letter
ready to merge

15 February 2008

«Patient_UR_number»

«title» «given_name» «surname»

Dear «given_name»

Thank you for attending the hospital today.
We are training new staff today and
apologise for any delays you might
experience. We will do our best to look
after you as quickly as possible.

Regards

Jane Smith

CEO

Step 5

The next step is to preview the letters (Fig 3.38). If something is wrong, go back (using the **Previous** link) and correct the letter.

Figure 3.38
Preview of a
letter produced
from Mail Merge

15 February 2008

300233

Mr Fred Smith

Dear Fred,

Thank you for attending the hospital today. We are training new
staff today and apologise for any delays you might experience. We
will do our best to look after you as quickly as possible.

Regards

Step 6

Finally, complete the mail merge. You can choose to go directly to **Print** or, if you want to make a final check, choose **Edit individual letters**.

3.1.7 Spelling and dictionaries – some tips

Word-processers provide some simple tools to assist in improving the quality of the documents produced. These include dictionary facilities.

Setting the language

If you look at the bottom of your Word window you should see an area that indicates the language/dictionary being used to check the document. In the document in Figure 3.39 it is English (Australia).

Figure 3.39
Dictionary being used

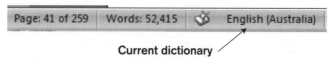

If you want to change the current dictionary you first need to decide if the change is for the whole document or just for the section you are currently working on. This type of change is usually for the entire document, in which case ensure that no text is selected, then double-click on the current dictionary area and the window in Figure 3.40 will appear. Choose the dictionary to be used for the document.

Figure 3.40
Dictionary selection dialog box

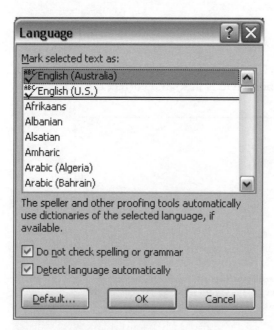

If you don't see the language area in the bottom bar:

- in Word 2007, go to **Review ➤ Set Language**
- in Word 2003, go to **Tools ➤ Language ➤ Set Language**.

If you only want part of a document to have a different language, e.g. a section of French, highlight the text you want to change, then set the language.

Autocorrect

To improve your typing a feature called Autocorrect is also provided as an option. Autocorrect takes a specific word entered and will always replace it with the 'correct' word.

One common autocorrection that can cause difficulties with healthcare documentation is EHR (which stands for Electronic Health Record). As originally set up, Word will change 'EHR' to 'her', because the table of corrections to be made indicates that EHR is a misspelling of her. To stop the computer doing this, remove this entry in the autocorrection table.

- In Word 2007, go to **Office Button ➤ Word Options** (at the bottom of the box that opens). Under **Proofing**, choose **AutoCorrect Options** to display the AutoCorrect dialog box.
- In Word 2003, go to **Tools ➤ AutoCorrect Options**.

This will display a window like that in Figure 3.41.

Figure 3.41
AutoCorrect options in Word 2007

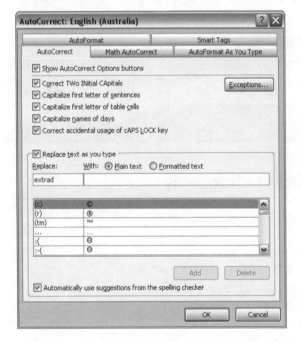

Look at the table near the bottom. If the values in the left-hand column are entered by you, they are automatically replaced by the values in the right-hand column. Try entering (c), and see what the program does. Now scroll down to 'ehr', select it and delete it.

This feature can be particularly useful if you have words you commonly mistype. Enter the mistyping in the 'Replace' section and type the correct word in the 'With' column. This can also be used to automatically expand abbreviations into full terms. You could enter 'eg' and have the system automatically expand this to 'for example'.

3.1.8   Mathematical equations

It is possible to insert properly laid-out mathematical equations in Word (and PowerPoint), by using the Equation Editor.

In Word 2007 this is automatically installed but if you are still using Word 2003, you may need to install it specially or ask your IT department to install it, as it is not normally installed as part of the Word 2003 package. It does not cost any more, as it simply involves turning on functionality that is available but not often used, but you will need your original installation CD.

To use Equation Editor:

- In Word 2007, go to the **Insert** ribbon, and in the **Symbols** section to the right choose **Equation**. You can choose from a set of standard equations or insert a new equation of your own. A box opens in the text, and the Equation Tools toolbar will appear.
- In Word 2003 (once installed), go to **Insert ➤ Object** and scroll down to select **Microsoft Equation 3.0**; click on **OK**. A box opens in the text, and the Equation toolbar will appear.

Figure 3.42
Equation tools
(Word 2007)

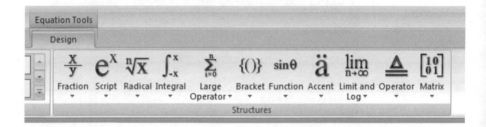

3.2   Using PowerPoint effectively

Learning objectives

When this section is completed you will be able to:
- open, close, create and save PowerPoint files
- insert a new slide, and chose its layout
- insert text and bullet lists
- insert charts and other graphics
- change the appearance of the slide show
- create simple animations
- create slide transitions
- create speakers notes
- print the presentation in formats suitable for different purposes.

PowerPoint (or a similar presentation package) is ideal if you need to present your information to a 'live' audience. Depending on the nature of the presentation, it is often appropriate to produce a handout for the audience. This can be as simple as a copy of your PowerPoint slides or, if you are using your presentation to introduce a large report, you might produce a short executive summary.

You can also create a presentation to run unattended. This can be useful if you are taking part in an organised event, or if you have access to information kiosks that can run presentations. The skills needed are a little different to those where the presenter will be presenting in person to an audience, and it is this latter method of presenting that we will discuss in this section. Some tips on designing PowerPoint for independent use are given in section 3.4.2.

3.2.1 Getting started

Presentation design

PowerPoint is the name of the presentation package in the Microsoft Office suite. Other packages are available to do the same job as PowerPoint, but the appearance and range of functions available will be different to those shown here.

The most important part of a presentation isn't the slides that you produce – it's the *information* that you are going to share. Remember, your presentation should help the audience to understand your message; it is not the message in itself. There's a well-known adage in public speaking: 'Tell them what you're going to say; say it; tell them what you've told them.' This holds true as a guideline for structuring your slide presentation.

It is easy to get carried away with the many effects that PowerPoint makes available; however, it is important to remember that *simplicity is generally best*. The presentation shouldn't have so many added bells and whistles that the audience becomes distracted by the presentation and overlooks your message. Some useful design hints to remember are:

1 Images can enhance the presentation of your information, but it is important that they are *relevant* to the content of the slide you put them on; otherwise you may confuse your audience.
2 A chart can display numerical or statistical information with much greater clarity than trying to describe it in words can achieve.
3 Words can blend into the background if the colours used are too close to each other. Different computer screens and projectors can display colours slightly differently, so something that looks just about okay on your computer might not work when shown through a projector.
4 Give each slide a title.
5 Design templates should complement the style and content of the presentation.
6 Use effects such as sounds and high-impact animations very sparingly.
7 Make sure that the font size used is large enough to be easily visible to the audience (for a lecture room around 28pt is a good basis, but think about the size of the audience, of the presentation room and of the projected image).

8 Use a simple, clear font, and keep it consistent across all of your slides.

9 Run the spellchecker!

10 If possible, get someone else to proofread your slides. It is very hard to spot your own mistakes, as you tend to read what you think should be there rather than what is actually there.

11 Don't take the text right up to the edge of the slide; keeping some space around the text makes the slide easier for people to read.

12 Don't try to write the whole presentation on the slides; you can use speaker's notes for yourself to help you remember what you plan to say.

13 Don't read the content of the slides to the audience; use summary points and expand on those as you talk.

Some PowerPoint hints and tips

- Having opened PowerPoint, the first thing to do to create your presentation is to make a title page and *save* the presentation. Most software programs are very stable and seldom crash while you are working on them, but technology isn't foolproof and is subject to external problems – a sudden power-cut could shut down your computer for you. It therefore makes sense to regularly save your work as you go, that way if the worst does happen you won't lose too much work. (This applies to all computer work, of course.)

  In PowerPoint we recommend saving your work after every slide. You can also set PowerPoint to automatically save your work in the background so that it can be auto-recovered if you have a problem. Do this through **Office Button ➤ PowerPoint Options ➤ Save** for PowerPoint 2007 and through **Tools ➤ Options ➤ Save** for PowerPoint 2003.

- If you are producing your PowerPoint for distribution rather than presenting it in person to an audience you can use the speaker's notes to add supporting information for the readers. You can also add audio to your files to help people follow them; this is covered in section 3.4.2.

How this section works

Worked examples 3.3 and 3.4

In this section, we initially explore the layout of the PowerPoint interface; then we move on to creating different types of slide. We suggest that you look at the example on the CD, *Example 3-3.ppt*, which shows different types of slide and animations. Initially, try copying the slides in the example. When you are confident about creating the individual slides, try creating a short presentation to share some information with colleagues.

We have also created a second example, *Example 3-4.ppt*, which shows you how *not* to do it. Each slide here contains examples and comments on some common mistakes that we see in student presentations.

3.2.2 Finding your way around

To create a PowerPoint presentation you need to first open the PowerPoint program. You can do this from the Start menu at the bottom left of your Windows screen.

Normal View layout
The main areas of the default opening setup are shown in Figure 3.43.

- **Screen View** options: PowerPoint opens in Normal View; see page 74 for information on the other options.
- The **Navigation** panel shows all the slides in the presentation. As you create new slides they will be added to the list here.
- **Speaker's notes**: discussed in section 3.2.6.
- **Main window**: this is where the slide that you are working on is open.

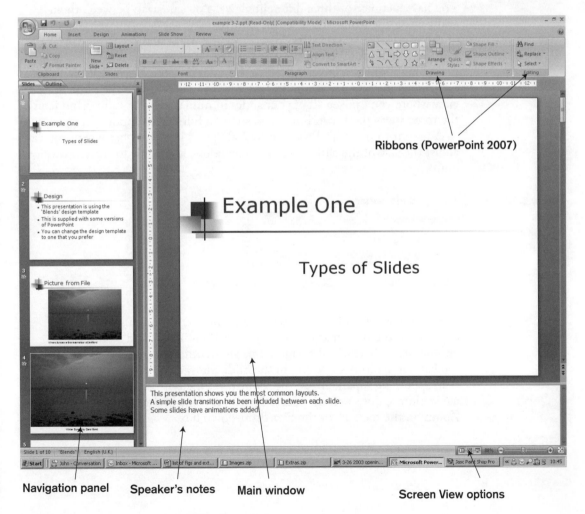

Figure 3.43 Default screen on opening PowerPoint

As with the other Microsoft Office programs, PowerPoint has tabs (and linked ribbons in the 2007 version). Many of the commands, such as **Office Button ➤ Save**, are the same. There are also some that are specific to PowerPoint; see Figure 3.44.

Insert slide elements, e.g. art, charts and sounds

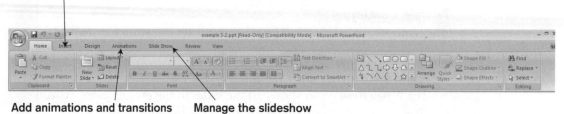

Add animations and transitions   Manage the slideshow

Figure 3.44 PowerPoint 2007 tabs

You have a choice of three different views. You can swap between them easily using the icons in the screen view panel at the bottom right-hand side of the window (Fig 3.45). In PowerPoint 2003, these three icons can be found at the bottom left of the PowerPoint window.

The highlighted icon at the left of these three is the Normal View – the one shown in the screenshot. The middle icon takes you to the Slide Sorter, a view where you can see all of your slides in miniature. The right-hand icon of the three starts the PowerPoint slideshow in full-screen mode.

Adjacent to these (in PowerPoint 2007 only) is a slider bar where you can adjust the size of the slide in the main window, and a 'Fit to current window' button.

Figure 3.45
Screen View
options in
PowerPoint 2007

Slide sorter

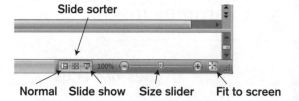

Normal   Slide show   Size slider   Fit to screen

The screen layout in PowerPoint 2003 is similar, although with toolbars rather than the ribbon at the top in PowerPoint 2007, and screen view options at the bottom, although items are in different places. On the toolbar, animations are found in the **Slide Show** drop-down menu rather than appearing separately on the toolbar. At the bottom of the screen, the navigation options are on the left-hand side. Size is altered using **View ➤ Zoom** on the toolbar, or the **Size** drop-down box.

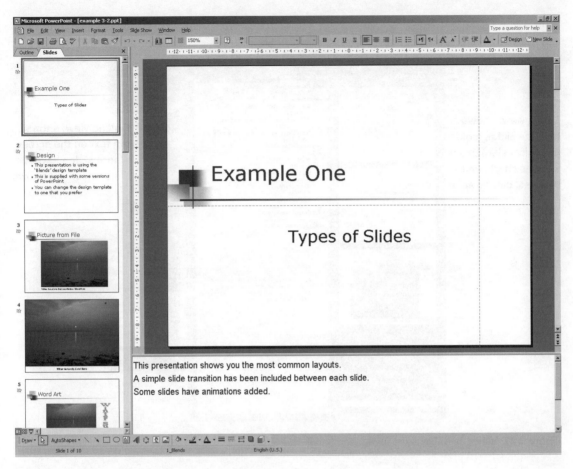

Figure 3.46 Layout differences in PowerPoint 2003

The Navigation panel in the left-hand column offers two different views of your slides. In Figure 3.47 (overleaf) they are shown side by side so that you can see the differences. In practice you can view one or the other, but not both.

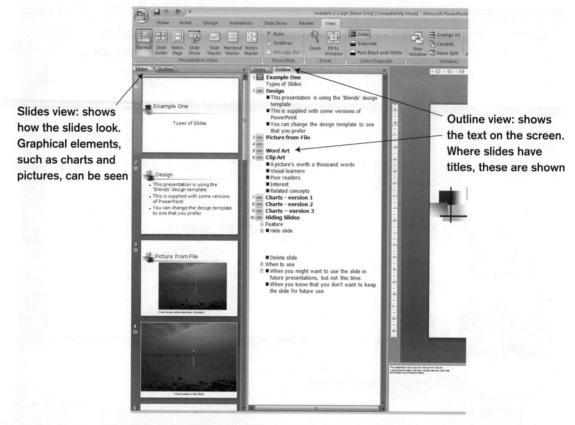

Slides view: shows how the slides look. Graphical elements, such as charts and pictures, can be seen

Outline view: shows the text on the screen. Where slides have titles, these are shown

Figure 3.47 Views available in the Navigation panel

Once you have created all your slides you can view them all at once (depending on the number of slides and the size of your computer screen) by using the Slide Sorter view (Fig 3.48).

As well as viewing all of your slides, in this view you can drag your slides to a different position in the presentation.

Right-clicking on a slide allows you to make changes to its layout. It also enables you to hide the slide. This means that it stays in your PowerPoint presentation, but does not appear in the slide show.

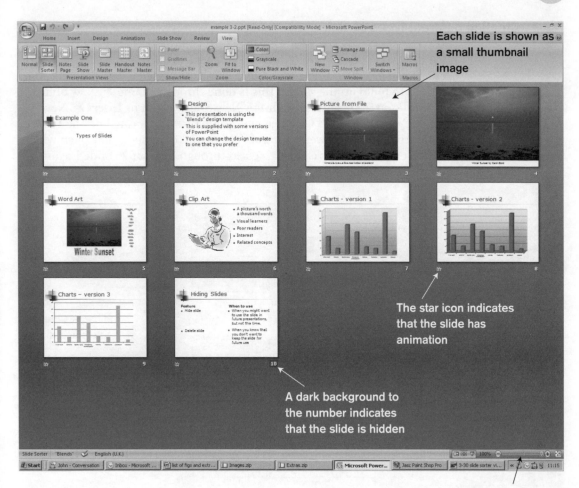

Figure 3.48 Slide Sorter view in PowerPoint 2007. The 2003 version is similar, though hidden slides are shown by the slide number being crossed out

Choosing the Slide Show option will start your slide show from the slide that is currently selected. You can navigate through the presentation one slide, or one element, at a time using the cursor keys on the keyboard or the mouse. If you want to move more than this, either forwards or backwards, a right-click will bring up a navigation menu. The 'Go to Slide' option here allows you to chose to open a slide navigator. This shows you the slide title, or the slide number if it does not have a title. You can use the ESC key to cancel the slide show at any time.

3.2.3   Creating different types of slide

Each time you open PowerPoint you can chose to open an existing presentation or create a new one. Once you have started a new presentation, you need to build up the slides. This is done through **Home ➤ New Slide** in PowerPoint 2007 and through the **New Slide** button or **Insert ➤ New Slide** in PowerPoint 2003. The layout options are also located on the **Home** ribbon (Fig 3.49) in PowerPoint 2007; in the 2003 version, they open when you insert a new slide or can be accessed through **Format ➤ Slide Layout**.

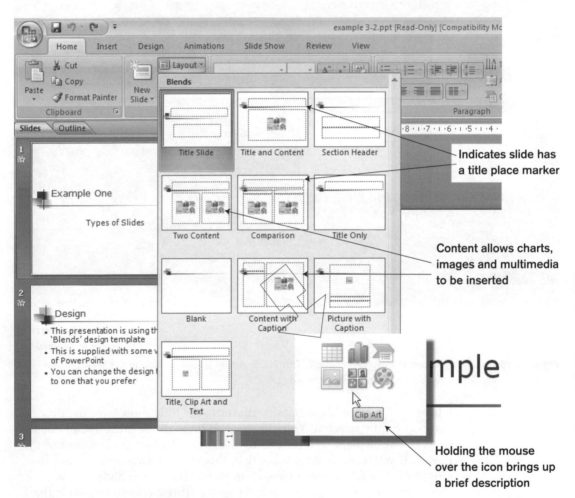

Figure 3.49 Slide layout presets in PowerPoint 2007

As well as various content and layout options, there is a blank slide option. This can be useful if the preset layouts don't have the various sections where you need them to be. Unless there is a good reason not to, always choose a layout with a slide title place marker, and use it. Titles are used in the navigation panel in Outline view, and in the Slide Show navigation screen, to help you find specific slides.

Worked examples 3.3 and 3.4 continued

Examples of each of the slides shown in Figure 3.49 are included in *Example 3-3.ppt* on the CD. As you read through this section look at the examples, and then try to create your own. The file *Example 3-4.ppt* has examples of how *not* to do things.

You have the flexibility to insert many different types of elements, including pictures, Clip Art, WordArt, charts and multimedia elements. Different elements can be combined on slides, but make sure you don't try to cram too much information onto one slide as this will make it difficult for your audience to know which part they should focus on.

Text and bullet-point lists

There are several preset layout options that include bullet-point lists. Think about which will best fit your information. The simplest is a single list; this can be seen on Slide 2 in *Example 3-3.ppt*. Other options include two columns of bullet points, which can be useful if you are making comparisons between two things (example on Slide 10). Or you might want a graphic on one side of the slide and a list of key points that relate to it on the other (example on Slide 6).

If you prefer a different symbol as your bullet, you can change these. It's best to change them across all slides, not just one, and this can be done on the Slide Master (see under section 3.2.4.).

Images and graphics

You can insert a variety of image types into your presentation.

- If you're working from a preset slide layout that includes image options, left-clicking the appropriate icon will open a context-sensitive dialog box.
- If you want to position an image on a blank slide you need to use **Insert**, and then chose the type of image you want to insert.
- If you want to use artistic effects on your text, you might want to look at 'WordArt'. As with any effect this should be used sparingly – on a word or two at most, not whole blocks of text (an example is shown in *Example 3-3.ppt*, Slide 5).
- If you have an image of your own that you want to use, perhaps a photograph that illustrates the point you are making, you can chose **Insert ➤ Picture** (PowerPoint 2007) or **Insert ➤ Picture ➤ From File** (PowerPoint 2003) and find the image on your hard drive or a CD. Remember that if you're using an image that you don't hold the copyright for, you need to check what restrictions there are on it, and that you have permission to use it for your presentation.

Clip Art

PowerPoint also has a collection of Clip Art that you can use. The collection includes cartoon-style graphics as well as photographic-style pictures.

Inserting Clip Art is done through **Insert ➤ Clip Art** (PowerPoint 2007) or **Insert ➤ Picture ➤ Clip Art** (PowerPoint 2003). This opens a new box in the right-hand panel (Fig 3.50) which can be used to search or browse the available Clip Art collections. Note that you can't actually open both of the drop-down boxes at the same time; you do one, then the other.

Figure 3.50
Clip Art panel

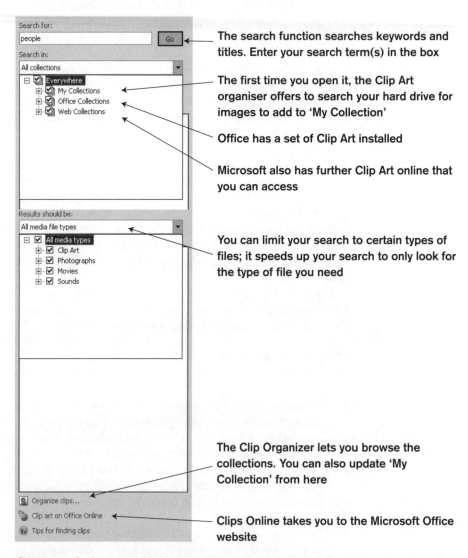

The search function searches keywords and titles. Enter your search term(s) in the box

The first time you open it, the Clip Art organiser offers to search your hard drive for images to add to 'My Collection'

Office has a set of Clip Art installed

Microsoft also has further Clip Art online that you can access

You can limit your search to certain types of files; it speeds up your search to only look for the type of file you need

The Clip Organizer lets you browse the collections. You can also update 'My Collection' from here

Clips Online takes you to the Microsoft Office website

Once you find a suitable image, insert it into your slide by either double-clicking it or dragging it across to your slide and dropping it.

Charts

As with most software programs, there is more than one way of doing something. We will look at two different ways of inserting graphs.

- One way is to create your chart in Excel (see Chapter 4, section 4.5.1) and then copy and paste it into PowerPoint. If you are doing this, please

also read the later section on PDF format.
- The other is to use the PowerPoint charting option, outlined below.

Note: make sure that you chose a chart style that is appropriate for your data. Chapter 4 (section 4.5.2) contains advice on choosing the right type of chart, and explains how to create charts from spreadsheets.

To insert a graph, first choose a preset slide layout that has an image of a chart on it (Fig 3.49).

- In PowerPoint 2007, use **Insert ➤ Chart** or left-click on the chart icon (Fig 3.51) on the slide layout.

Figure 3.51
Insert Chart icon

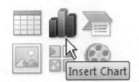

This opens a new box offering you a wide range of chart styles (Fig 3.52).

Figure 3.52
Chart options

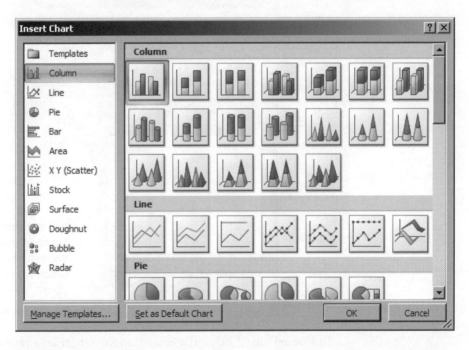

Left-click on your chosen chart style and choose OK; an Excel spreadsheet will open and your PowerPoint slide will automatically be reduced in size so that both the Excel spreadsheet and the PowerPoint slide are open on your screen.

You will see that there is already some sample data in the spreadsheet which are graphed on the chart. You can make the Excel data area larger or smaller to accommodate your data (Fig 3.53). As you start to replace the sample data with your own data the chart automatically updates itself with the new data. You can add and delete rows and columns in the spreadsheet. The tabs/ribbons also allow you to edit the chart.

Figure 3.53
Editing Chart
Data

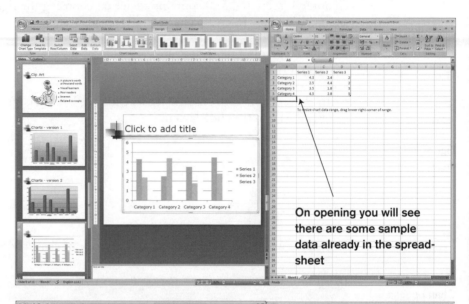

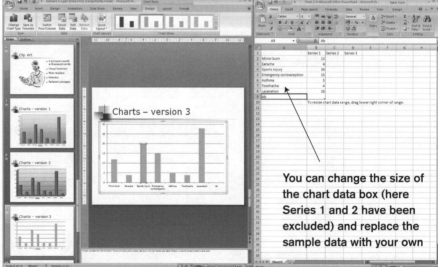

• In PowerPoint 2003, left-clicking on the Chart icon immediately pastes a sample chart into your slide, along with a small Excel-type datasheet window containing the sample data (Fig 3.54). Right-click in the main chart area and choose **Chart Options** to see a range of other types of chart to choose from. Change the sample data in the datasheet to your own data, and the chart will update.

Figure 3.54
Creating a chart
in PowerPoint
2003

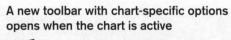
A new toolbar with chart-specific options opens when the chart is active

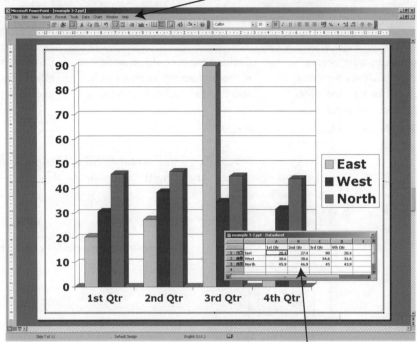

The spreadsheet opens in this small window. You can drag it around the screen and resize it if necessary

If you create a chart in PowerPoint (or import it from Excel as a chart), you can animate it at the individual column level rather than at the complete chart level – which is the only option if you insert it as an image. This is discussed further in section 3.2.5. Have a look at *Example 3-3.ppt*, slides 7, 8 and 9 to see the differences.

3.2.4 Enhancing slide appearance

There are several things you can do to enhance the appearance of your presentation:

- apply a Slide Design theme or template
- edit the Master Slide to set overall preferences
- use animations and transitions.

Design themes and templates
PowerPoint offers you a range of design templates and colour schemes. You need to choose a template that will both complement the content of your presentation and appeal to your target audience.
- In PowerPoint 2007, you can access the template panel through the **Design** ribbon (Fig 3.55).

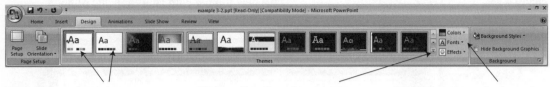

Moving your cursor across
the designs shows how that
design will look on the slide
open in the main window

Clicking the drop-down arrow
at the bottom will open a box to
show all the available options

Colour schemes, fonts and
effects can be changed within
each design

Figure 3.55 Design ribbon in PowerPoint 2007

• In PowerPoint 2003, go to **Format ➤ Slide Design,** and a panel of
options will appear at the right-hand side.

Figure 3.56
Slide design in
PowerPoint 2003

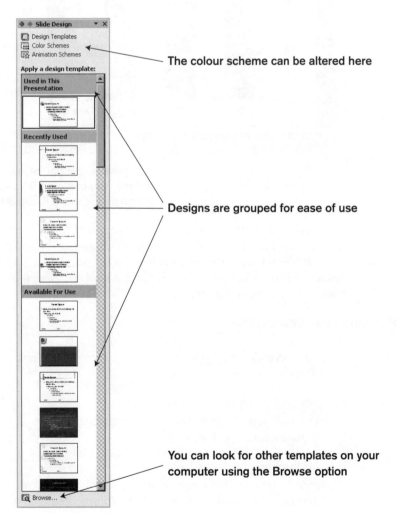

The colour scheme can be altered here

Designs are grouped for ease of use

You can look for other templates on your
computer using the Browse option

Master Slides

Your audience will find your presentation easier to view if you make sure
that all the visual elements, such as font type and size, are consistent across
all your slides. You can do this by editing the default settings on the Slide
Master.

- In PowerPoint 2007, go to **View ➤ Slide Master**.
- In PowerPoint 2003, go to **View ➤ Master ➤ Slide Master**.

Each type of slide you have used in your presentation is shown (Fig 3.57),
and you can edit each element.

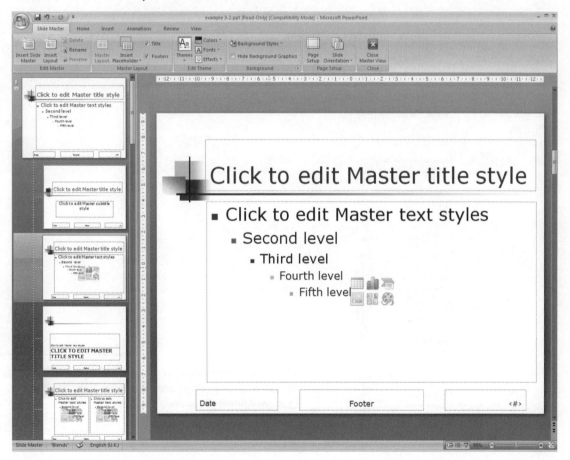

Figure 3.57 Slide Master

3.2.5 Animations and transitions

Animations are movement effects added to a single slide. Transitions are
effects used when moving from one slide to the next. In PowerPoint 2007
these are available in the **Animations** tab, and in PowerPoint 2003 via the
Slide Show menu item.

Animations

These are used to build up your slide by bringing in the various elements within it, to highlight the particular point you are speaking about. For example, you can bring the points in a bullet list in one at a time, rather than having them all visible on the slide when you open it.

You have the choice of using a preset animation scheme or creating a custom one (Figs 3.58 and 3.59).

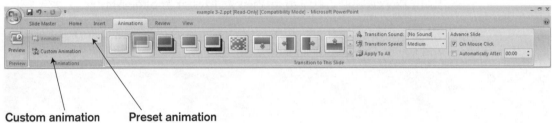

Custom animation   **Preset animation**

Figure 3.58 Animation ribbon in PowerPoint 2007

Figure 3.59
Animation
schemes in
PowerPoint 2003

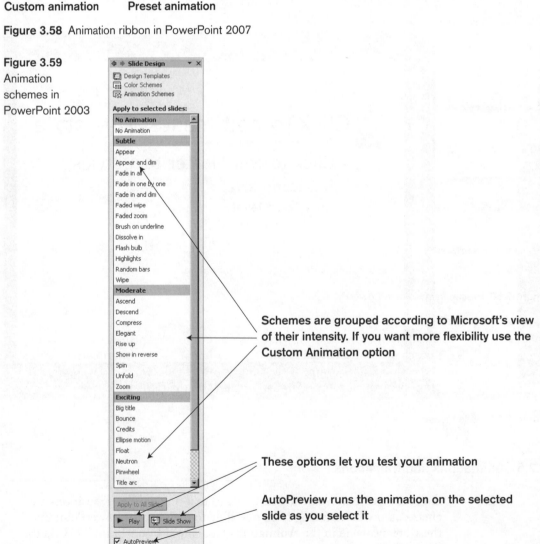

Schemes are grouped according to Microsoft's view of their intensity. If you want more flexibility use the Custom Animation option

These options let you test your animation

AutoPreview runs the animation on the selected slide as you select it

In PowerPoint 2007, you cannot select 'Animate' until you have selected the area on the slide that you want to animate. Once this is done, you can select a preset animation (Fig 3.60). You will see that the text selected for animation is shown with a box around it.

In PowerPoint 2003, each animation scheme is applied automatically to each of the elements on the slide.

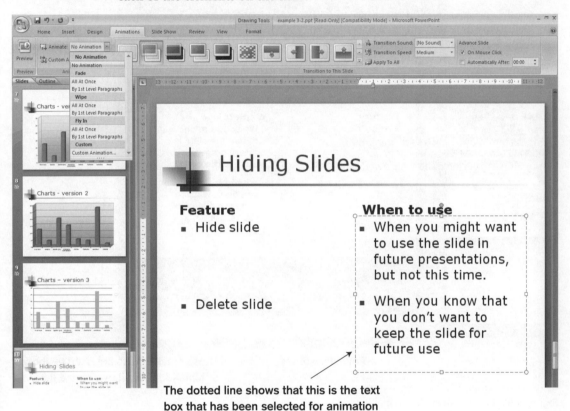

The dotted line shows that this is the text box that has been selected for animation

Figure 3.60 Preset animations in PowerPoint 2007

If you want more control, you can structure your own animations. To do this, choose the **Custom Animation** option on the **Animations** ribbon in PowerPoint 2007 or under the **Slide Show** menu item in PowerPoint 2003. This opens the Custom Animation panel on the right-hand side of your screen (Fig 3.61).

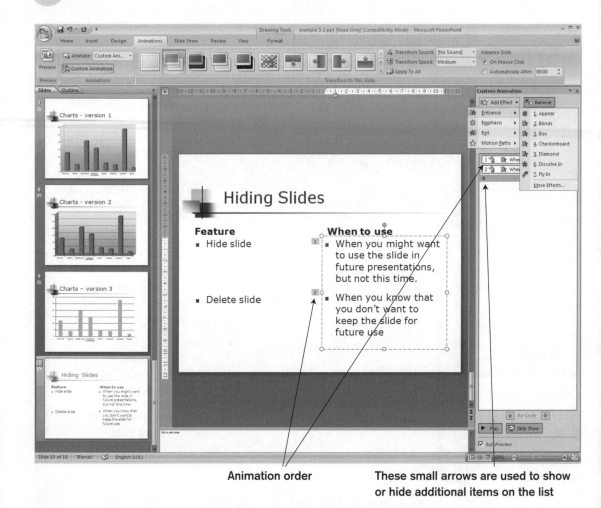

Animation order

These small arrows are used to show or hide additional items on the list

Figure 3.61 Custom Animation panel

- The numbers on the left-hand side of each bullet point on the slide represent the order that they will be brought onto the slide in the presentation. You can change the order by selecting a bullet point (or other element) in the right-hand panel and using the up and down arrows near the bottom of the panel.
- The effects are grouped according to type. If you select **More Effects** at the bottom of the effects submenu, a new box opens with all of the available effects grouped according to intensity (Fig 3.62).

Figure 3.62
The full range of
animation effects

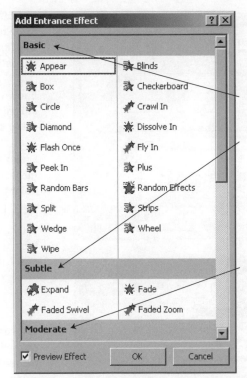

'Basic' and 'Subtle' effects are
best for regular use, but be
consistent throughout your
presentation. Don't keep changing
from one style to another

'Moderate' can add impact, but
use very sparingly

'Exciting' can have people
watching what the PowerPoint
software can do rather than
focusing on what it is that you're
trying to say

- Once you have added an effect you can edit each item individually
  (Fig 3.63).

Figure 3.63
Custom
Animation
settings

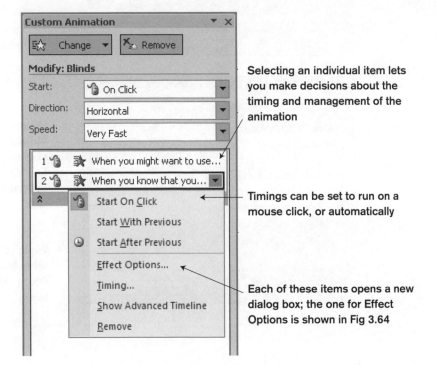

Selecting an individual item lets
you make decisions about the
timing and management of the
animation

Timings can be set to run on a
mouse click, or automatically

Each of these items opens a new
dialog box; the one for Effect
Options is shown in Fig 3.64

Figure 3.64
Animation effects

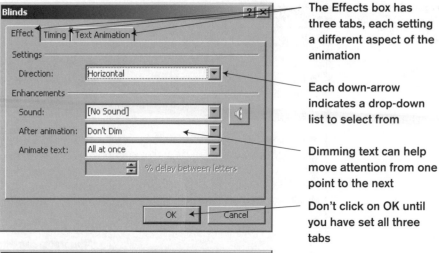

The Effects box has three tabs, each setting a different aspect of the animation

Each down-arrow indicates a drop-down list to select from

Dimming text can help move attention from one point to the next

Don't click on OK until you have set all three tabs

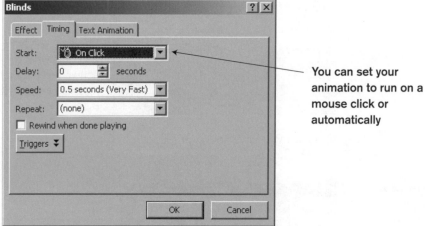

You can set your animation to run on a mouse click or automatically

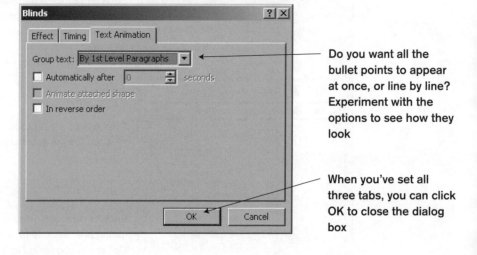

Do you want all the bullet points to appear at once, or line by line? Experiment with the options to see how they look

When you've set all three tabs, you can click OK to close the dialog box

- You have the option of setting your animations to progress on a mouse click, or on set timings. If you are doing a live presentation, you have much more control if you advance on a mouse click. However much you practise, you may not speak at the same speed when doing the presentation for real. A mouse click also allows you the flexibility of pausing if your audience has any questions about the point you are making, or if any interruption happens.
- If you have created a chart in PowerPoint (see section 3.2.3) or pasted one in from Excel *as a chart object*, you can fully animate it by selecting your animation to operate 'By Element in Series'. This can be done through **Custom Animation**. The third tab on the Animation Effects box (Fig 3.64) will read **Chart Animation** rather than Text Animation, and will give you the option to animate by series or by category. Try both and see which works best for your chart.

  In PowerPoint 2007 you can also animate your chart directly from the Animations ribbon (Fig 3.65).

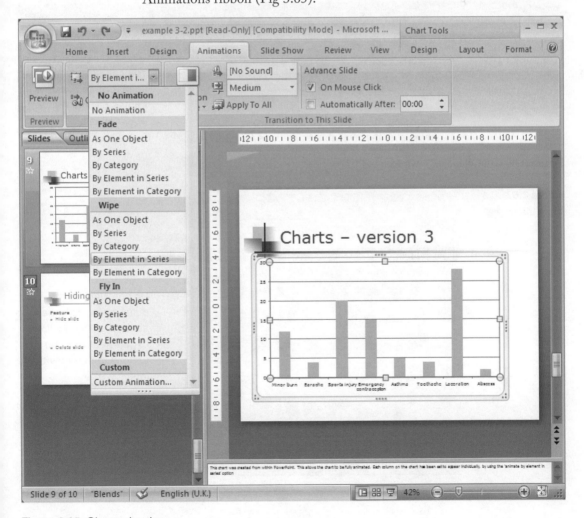

Figure 3.65 Chart animation

Quick hint

If you have created a chart previously and come back to animate it later, you may find that the third tab isn't showing. If this happens, click out of the Chart Animation box, double-click on the chart to select it and then re-open the animation options.

As you have seen, animations have many variables that you can set. Some variables work best with some animations. For example, bringing a short heading in one word (or even one letter) at a time may add impact, whereas bringing in a slide of bullet points a single word at a time can be very tedious for the audience.

Transitions

Transitions can enable you to glide from one slide to another in style. Transitions are accessed through the **Animations** tab in PowerPoint 2007 (Fig 3.66) and through the **Slide Show** menu item in PowerPoint 2003 (Fig 3.68).

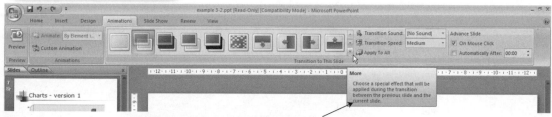

Choosing the More drop-down arrow
reveals all the available transitions (Fig 3.67)

Figure 3.66 Transitions in PowerPoint 2007

Figure 3.67
More transitions

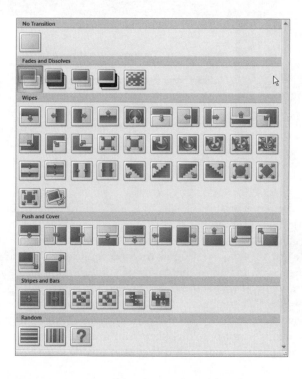

Figure 3.68
Slide Transition
options in
PowerPoint 2003

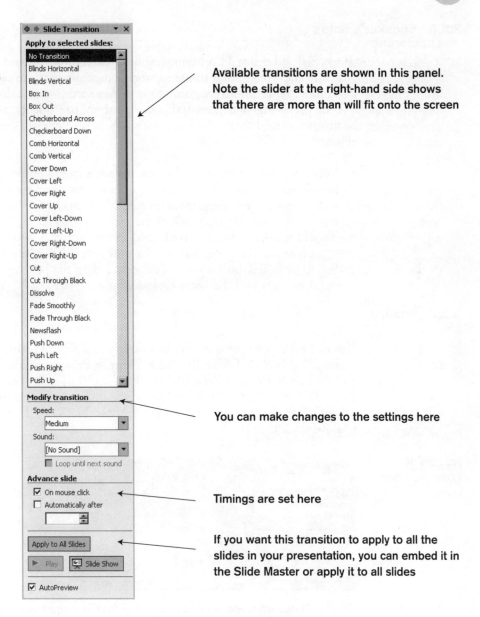

Available transitions are shown in this panel.
Note the slider at the right-hand side shows
that there are more than will fit onto the screen

You can make changes to the settings here

Timings are set here

If you want this transition to apply to all the
slides in your presentation, you can embed it in
the Slide Master or apply it to all slides

As with all effects, it is important to be consistent across all of your
presentation, and remember that subtlety is generally best.

If possible, check what version of PowerPoint the presentation equipment
has. If it's not the same version as the one you used to prepare your
presentation, you may find that some of your animations are not compatible
and will not run. If this is the case, the text (or chart) will appear on the slide
at the outset rather than according to the steps you had planned. You may be
able to have a run-through on the presentation equipment to check before
you start; if this is not possible, keep your animations simple and think about
how the presentation will look if they don't work.

3.2.6   Speaker's notes

The actual slides should contain your key points only. Thus, it can be useful to create additional notes to use as an aide memoir to make sure that you don't forget what you were going to say. These are also useful to include if you are preparing your presentation to hand out to students, as they will be able to remind themselves of what you said (rather than over-filling the slides).

- When working with printed notes, it's advisable to fasten them together loosely so that you can turn the pages easily but can't get them out of order – even if you drop them. A single hole in the top left-hand corner linked by a treasury tag works well.
- To add speaker's notes to your slide, move your cursor to the notes section below the slide, and type in your notes. If you want more of the box to be visible on the screen, click-and-drag the bar that divides the main window and the notes area to adjust the size.

3.2.7   Printing

You can print your presentation in a variety of different formats. Open the **Print** dialog box via **Office Button ➤ Print ➤ Print** in PowerPoint 2007 and via **File ➤ Print** in PowerPoint 2003 (or CRTL-P in both versions). You may notice that the top sections of the dialog box are similar to those in other Office applications. The bottom section (Fig 3.69), however, is unique to PowerPoint.

Figure 3.69
PowerPoint print features

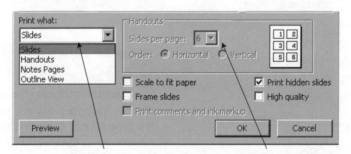

Chose *what* you want to print   This is greyed out (inactive) until
                                        'Handouts' are selected in **Print what**

Printing slides
Slides will print as one slide per page. If the paper is not the same size as the slide, use **Scale to fit paper** to force it to fit. You can choose whether to have a frame around your slides or not.

Printing handouts
By default the handout layout is set to six slides per page, although (as shown in Figure 3.70) there are several other options. Other than the three slides per page option, the only difference is the number of slides per page, and thus their size. Three slides per page is, however, on a different layout to all of the

other options. As can be seen in the small box, the slides are placed on the left-hand side of the page, with lines next to them. This layout is particularly useful if you think people may want to take notes during your presentation.

Figure 3.70
Printing handouts

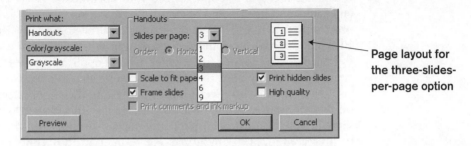

Page layout for the three-slides-per-page option

Printing speaker's notes

Selecting 'Notes Pages' under **Print what** will include your speaker's notes on the same page as the relevant slide. As with printing slides, this prints one slide (plus notes) per page.

3.3 PDF format

Learning objectives

By the end of this section you will:

- know what a PDF file is
- know some reasons why you may want to share information in the PDF format
- understand how PDFs can contribute to confidentiality
- know how to create a PDF file.

3.3.1 Why use PDF?

As a user of information, you're likely to have some experience of PDF documents. Many organisations (e.g. the UK's National Health Service, NHS) produce their policy documents in the PDF format for anyone to download from their websites. Academic journals also frequently offer their papers in this way.

In this section we will look at *why* you might want to create a PDF version of your presentation. Spreadsheets, Word documents and PowerPoint-style presentations can all be converted into PDFs.

PDF is short for portable document format. This was created by Adobe, who also produce a free programme, Adobe Reader, to open and read PDF files. This is not the only programme that will do this; Macintosh users will find that their Preview programme can handle PDFs, and there are others available from both open-source and commercial providers.

One advantage of turning your document into a PDF is that doesn't matter what type of computer or operating system your readers are using – there is software available to open PDFs for all the main systems. PDFs thus make it easy for people to read your documents. Fonts/typefaces, special characters and images and objects can often 'drop out' of a document or presentation between different versions of Office programs. If you create a PDF instead, this locks in the information in the form you want it displayed.

It also doesn't matter from which type of application the PDF has been created; users only need the free reader to be able to open your PDF file. If you send someone a PowerPoint presentation, they either need PowerPoint on their computer or you need to package it with a PowerPoint viewer. The same is true for most commercial file formats – they need the program they were created in, or a compatible one, to open it. PDFs only need a reader, such as the one made freely available by Adobe.

Another very important reason for using PDFs is the added security that it gives your document. The importance of data security was discussed in the *Introduction* chapter. Even with the best of intentions, however, it is possible to breach patient confidentiality by accident or, more accurately, owing to a lack of awareness and understanding, as Exercise 3.5 below will show.

If you want to put documents on the Internet, PDF format is ideal, as it makes it easy for your audience to open the files, and is a more secure way maintaining the integrity of shared files than some other formats. PDF files also tend to be much smaller (fewer KB) than the source files (especially if you compress them for the Internet) and therefore are quicker and cheaper to send or post electronically. (KB = kilobyte = 1000 bytes. A byte is a piece of data, such as the letter A.)

Example 3.5

Consider this case study, which unfortunately really did happen in a UK NHS Trust. A manager was required to produce a report on the use of a call centre service for the trust's board at short notice. The patient record system in use couldn't produce the information in the format that was needed, so the data were cut and pasted into Excel. A chart was made from that, and inserted into a Word document.

Before we move onto what happened next, try this out for yourself, in Exercise 3.5.

EXERCISE 3.5

1 Open the Excel spreadsheet *Confidential data.xls* on the CD and scroll down Sheet 1 until you can see the chart. Select the chart and copy it (CTRL-C).

2 Now open the Word document *Board Report.doc* and do a special paste of the chart, just underneath where it says 'Insert Chart Here'. To do this:

❐ In Word 2007, **Paste** is in the **Home** tab. Under the Paste icon you will see a drop-down arrow. Selecting this will give you the choice to do a simple paste or to chose **Paste Special**. Chose this, and a new dialog box will open with various ways of pasting the chart into your Word file.

❐ In Word 2003, go to **Edit ➤ Paste Special** to get a Paste Special dialog box.

3 Select 'Microsoft Office Excel Chart Object' and left-click on OK to insert the chart into your document. Close the Excel spreadsheet.

4 Save the Word document as *Board Report with chart.doc*.

5 Now re-open *Board Report with chart.doc*, and double-click on the chart.

Example 3.5 continued

As you've just found, this copy and paste hasn't *only* copied across the chart, but it has also copied across *all* of the underlying data, including elements that can't be seen in the chart. This is exactly what happened with the chart included in the board report.

When copying and pasting charts between different Office applications, you thus need to take great care to know whether you have inserted a chart (or spreadsheet) object or an *image* of it. You should also remember that data should be anonymised before it is used for secondary purposes.

Example 3.5 continued

The final production stage for trust board papers was to convert them to PDFs. This stage was missed out because of the last-minute rush to get the papers circulated prior to the meeting.

These papers were sent to quite a lot of people, not only board members, but also the local press and others. In all they were sent to 35 people, and placed on the trust's website for a time.

The result of this was that the confidential information of 92 people, including names, addresses, telephone numbers and the reason why they had called the out-of-hours centre, was made publicly available. An inquiry identified that the people who had produced the report hadn't realised that the data were embedded in the chart.

The final stage of preparing the board papers *should* have been converting the document to a PDF; however, it appears that those involved hadn't realised the importance of this stage.

Converting to a PDF effectively locks the document off from underlying data. It's a bit like taking a photocopy rather than sending the original. Open the document *Trust Board Report.pdf* document on the CD. Try double-clicking on the chart there, and you'll see that you can't open it.

As well as locking off embedded data, creating a PDF means that people can't easily make changes to your document; another important reason for using this format. Depending on the software used to produce the PDF, you can stop people copying sections of the text.

3.3.3 Producing PDFs

Having given reasons for converting a document into a PDF file, the next question is *how*.

As well as the freely available viewer, Adobe produce Acrobat which is a very comprehensive program for converting a multitude of file formats to PDFs. It also offers a range of additional features, such as digital signatures, collaboration tools, and even sticky notes if you want to add your own comments as you read a document. Needless to say, as a commercial programme this is quite an expensive piece of software. If you just want to convert documents to PDF, rather than access all the other functions, you have some cheaper alternatives.

- In Office 2007 or on a Macintosh, you have the option of 'printing' your document to the PDF format without needing to download or buy any additional programmes. Select print in the usual way (**File ➤ Print** or CTRL-P), and look at the bottom of the **Print** dialog box. Here you'll see a range of options for saving as a PDF (Fig 3.71). Make sure the filename you choose to save to has the .pdf extension.

Figure 3.71 Print to PDF options for a Macintosh

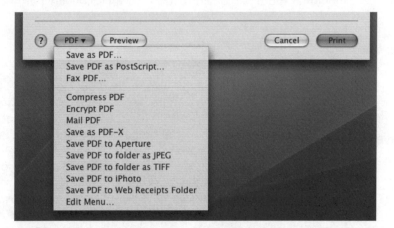

- Alternatively, the cheapest way of converting a document to PDF is to use a free program such as the OpenOffice suite of programmes. This is an open-source suite of Office-style programmes. 'Open source' means that the developers make the program code freely available; the Open Source Initative's website (www.opensource.org) gives more information if you are interested in the open-source movement. OpenOffice is available free of charge from www.openoffice.org. OpenOffice can open documents created in Microsoft Office. It can also save documents as PDF files, through the **Save As** menu.

3.3.3 Accessibility issues

Adobe Reader offers several useful features for people who have problems reading information. As well as being compatible with text readers such as the Kurzweil system, Adobe Reader has its own **Read Out Loud** function included, accessed through the **View** menu.

After creating a PDF document you check for accessibility problems by opening it in Adobe Reader and running its **Accessibility Quick Check** option, found under the **Document** menu.

3.4 The Internet

Learning objectives

When this section is completed you will be able to:
- know some ways of sharing information on the Internet
- have explored blogs and wikis
- have considered preparing PowerPoint for use on the Internet.

The Internet is a good way of sharing information when you do not know who the audience is. It enables you to make your information available to a wide range of people. This can create challenges for you in deciding how to best present your information, as the audience may be international and may have varying levels of understanding.

It's best for you to decide who you really want to read your web pages, and present your information in the way you think will work best for them.

Make sure you treat all personal information as confidential, and respect other people's intellectual property and copyright.

3.4.1 Ways to use the Internet

If you want to share the information that you have created with an anonymous group of people, such as 'patients' or 'healthcare professionals', then you need to find a way of putting your information in the public domain in a place that they are likely to find it.

The Internet is one place that many people go. In the UK the Office of National Statistics[1] reported that 61% of households had access to the Internet in 2007. Only 27% of people said they never used the Internet. Although the over-65s had the lowest use of any age group, with 71% saying they didn't use it, this group is growing the most rapidly. Data from the Australian Bureau of Statistics[2] show a similar picture. In 2006–07, 64% of Australian households had an Internet connection at home.

Some organisations, especially larger ones, have their own mini-Internet, called an Intranet. This uses the same technology as the Internet but its use is restricted to computers on the organisation's network. Sometimes people outside of the physical Intranet network may be able to access it through a password system.

Although we talk about 'the Internet' as a generic term, the Internet is actually the various hardware components that support a range of different software-driven services, such as the World Wide Web (www or Web) with its blogs and wikis, file transfer, online chat and email.

Email is only of use if you know the email address of the person you are sending something to. Even then, email should only be used if you know, or have good reason to believe, that the person won't mind receiving the information from you. Sending unsolicited emails to large lists of people is called spamming. You should avoid doing this for several reasons: it generally annoys the people receiving it; in some countries it is illegal; and it will often result in your email address being blocked by commercial email filtering systems. Even if you are trying to send an email across just a single organisation, you may well find that the email administrator has blocked the ability to send an email to 'all'. People have to identify the individuals or groups who need the information rather using than the blanket approach of sending it to everyone.

If you don't know the actual people who will be interested in your information, then the Web is probably the best option. There are three main ways of using the Web:

* as part of an existing website
* a wiki
* a blog.

Website

A Web page can be on the Internet or on an Intranet. One big advantage of being included in a larger site is that search engines are much more likely to find your information than if you have your own personal, very small site. How to set a website up from scratch is beyond the scope of this book; however, if you have access to an existing website there are several ways of presenting your information through it.

* One is to ask the website manager to post a PDF file on the site for you (see the section above for how to create a PDF file).
  Another is to provide the website manager with a Web page, or two. Ask them what format they would like the information in.

* Microsoft Office 2003 applications contain the function **Save File As Web Page**, while Word 2007 can save a Word document as a blog post (see over for more about blogs). This is done through the **Publish** option on the Office Button.

> **Quick hint**
>
> In Excel, you have the option of saving a single worksheet or the complete workbook. Remember to check all the worksheets very carefully for any confidential information (which may be hidden) before you decide to save the complete workbook to be placed on a website.

Blogs

Blog is short for a Web log – an online diary where you can record events and share information. One disadvantage of creating a blog to share your information is that your readers (or potential readers) will expect it to be dynamic, with regular new entries. If that isn't what you need for your information, or your audience, try looking at the next section on wikis. These have many things in common with blogs:

- they both require very little knowledge to set them up (if using one of the many free online versions)
- they are interactive, although membership may be required to be able to post (add information)
- most can be set to let the owner know when someone has made a post on the site
- pages can be archived.

The main difference is that blogs are more time-orientated than wikis, because they need regular updating to retain the dynamic aspect.

As with just about all Web tools, if you have your own website there is open-source software available to set up your own blog there.

If you don't have a website, or the technical skills, to set up your own blog you can use an online blogging service to create one. Any search engine will find blog sites. A well-known one is Blogger (www.blogger.com), owned by Google. As an example we've set up a blog called 'HEALTH-DATA' on Blogger. This can be viewed at http://health-data.blogspot.com.

The process of setting up a blog at blogger is very easy. The homepage offers you the option of creating a blog (Fig 3.72).

Figure 3.72
Blogger's home page

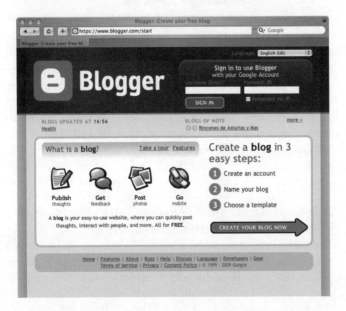

Once you've clicked on the 'Create your blog now' button and created a Google account if you didn't already have one, on-screen support takes you through the steps of naming your blog and deciding how you would like it to look. The final step is to create the first page of your blog, and publish it (Fig 3.73).

Figure 3.73
Publish your first blogger post

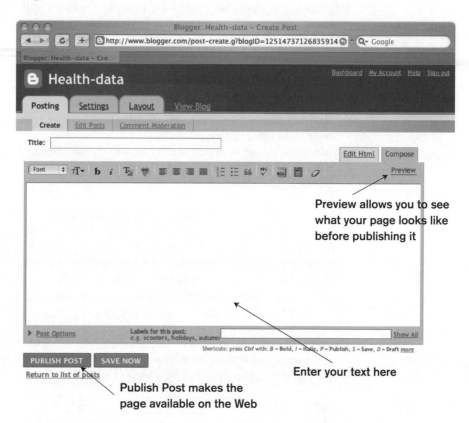

Preview allows you to see what your page looks like before publishing it

Enter your text here

Publish Post makes the page available on the Web

Wikis

Wikis are named after the Hawaiian word *wiki*, meaning fast. A wiki is simply software that allows users to create a Web page quickly and easily. A feature of a wiki page as opposed to other Web pages is that people can collaborate through them. You can post your information on your wiki, and invite others to either edit your posts, or add their own comments. Depending on the information that you are sharing, you may want to limit other people's ability to alter it.

It is possible to set up your own wiki; there are two main ways of doing this.

- One is to establish your own wiki service. This generally needs access to a Web server, and some technical knowledge.
- The other is to use a service such as Wikispaces (www.wikispaces.com), which offers both a free wiki and a paid-for service. As with many free online services, there are some restrictions: in this case you can't keep your wiki private, although you *can* limit who can edit it. Adverts may also be displayed on your page. The paid-for service does not have these limitations.

Before you sign up to any online services, free or paid for, it is sensible to check out their privacy policy. Are they going to keep your email address private; who will be able to see the information you provide on sign-up? Wikispaces (for example) assures users that:

we don't spam, we don't sell your personal information, and you can opt-out of all emails sent by our site.

Wikispaces offers a tutorial to new users that you can access once you have set up your wiki space. We've set up a test wiki there, where you can try editing a wiki page: http://health-data.wikispaces.com (Fig 3.74).

Figure 3.74
Wikispaces page

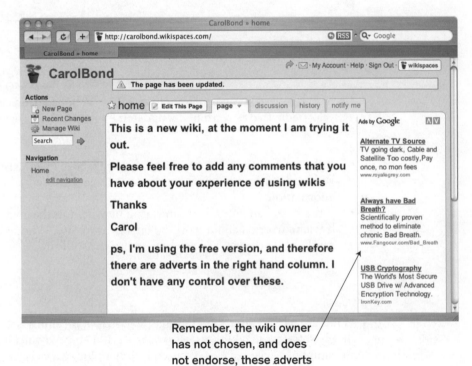

To use the wiki, click on **Join this Space**. You will be asked to sign in, or to join Wikispaces first if not already a member. Once you have done that, you can ask to join the health-data wiki (Fig 3.75). When asking to join, you need to mention the title of this book in your request.

Figure 3.75 Join
health-data wiki

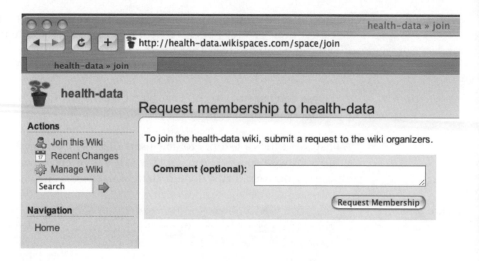

Perhaps the best-known collaborative wiki is Wikipedia, an online encyclopaedia that is continually updated by its user base (www.wikipedia.org).

- If the information that you want to share relates to an existing entry in Wikipedia, you can edit the entry to include the essential points in your information.
- If there isn't an entry, you can start a new item in the encyclopedia.
- If you're worried about working on a live website, Wikipedia offers you a 'sandbox' where you can see how to use the software.

EXERCISE 3.6

Go to Wikipedia now, and have a play in the sandbox. The URL for the English welcome page is http://en.wikipedia.org/wiki/Main_Page (Fig 3.76). At the top, underneath 'Welcome to Wikipedia' you'll see the tagline 'the free encyclopedia that anyone can edit.'

Figure 3.76
Wikipeda
home page

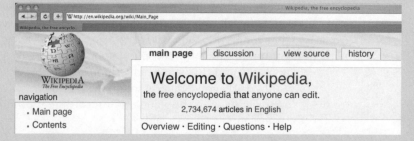

If you click on the text 'anyone can edit' you will be taken to a page that introduces editing Wikipedia. This page links to the sandbox.

3.4.2   PowerPoint and the Internet

If you want to share your PowerPoint presentation over the Internet, you have several options.

• It can be uploaded to the Web as a PowerPoint file. Different versions of PowerPoint have different levels of functionality, and some earlier versions may not be able to run the animations and transitions that you have used. People will need either PowerPoint, a compatible programme, or a PowerPoint viewer to be able to open and view the file.
• You can save it as a PDF document. This doesn't enable people to see it as a slideshow with animations or other enhancements, but it does mean people who don't have PowerPoint can usually open it without any problems. See the section on PDFs for more information about this option.
• You can save it as a Web page. PowerPoint takes care of the coding into html format ready for the Web, and produces a main Web page plus a folder with everything that is necessary for the presentation to be opened by a Web browser. All you need to do is upload the htm or html file and the folder, or pass them to your website manager who will be able to do that for you. (html stands for hypertext markup language, the special program language used on the Internet, particularly for Web page representation.)

If you are uploading a presentation, you need to take into account that the reader will only have your slides to read. This is usually not enough by itself. In a live presentation you supply *additional* information in person. There are a couple of things that you can do to replace your input.

• One is to use the speaker's notes section to add additional information.
• The other is to record a soundtrack to go with each slide so that your audience still gets to hear what you would have said.

Adding a soundtrack

PowerPoint makes the option of adding a soundtrack very easy to do. The hardest thing is working out what to say. We recommend writing yourself a script, or at least notes of what you want to say. Practise saying the text once or twice so that you are comfortable with it before you record it. You can add the soundtrack one slide at a time, and if you're not happy with the recording you can delete it and do it again.

If your computer has an inbuilt microphone this may be adequate for the task, or you might find that you need a slightly more powerful external one to capture sufficiently good-quality sound. Experiment with what you've got to see if you're happy with the standard of recording it produces.

To add your soundtrack to a slide:

• Select the slide that you want to add the sound to.
• Go to **Insert ➤ Sound ➤ Record Sound** (in PowerPoint 2007) or to **Insert ➤ Movies and Sounds ➤ Record Sound** in PowerPoint 2003. The dialog box shown in Figure 3.77 will open.

- The first thing to do is to name your sound clip; by default PowerPoint offers you 'Recorded Sound' as a name. We prefer to change this to the slide number that the clip relates to.
- Then it's simply a case of hitting the record button, saying your text and then stopping the recording with the stop button.

Figure 3.77
Record Sound
dialogue box

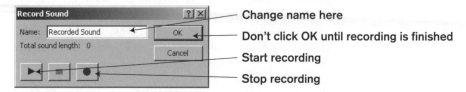

When you click on OK the Record Sound dialog box will close, and a small speaker icon will be placed on your slide. This shows that the audio clip is now embedded in the slide. You can move this to wherever you want it to be, and can resize it using the white dot on the corners.

You can then set how you want the soundtrack to play using the animation settings that we used in section 3.2.5. See Figure 3.78.

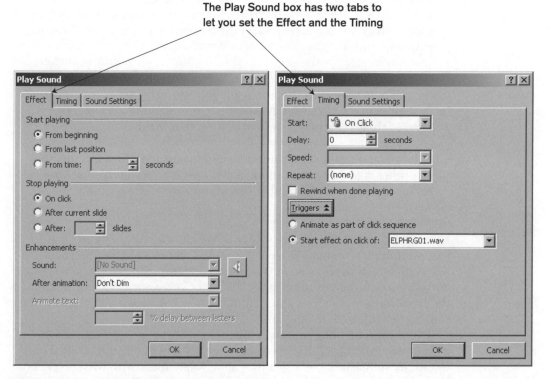

Figure 3.78 Animating sound clips in PowerPoint

You will need to set each parameter according to your sound clip, and your presentation. Once you have organised the sound clips, check how long they last and make sure that your other animations work with the sound. After you have set the effects, make sure that you run the show to see if the effects have worked as you wanted.

3.4.3 Accessibility issues on the Internet

Whatever format you chose for presenting your information, you want all of your intended audience to be able to access it. The layout and structure of the presentation is crucial. There are some things that you can inadvertently do that will make it more difficult for some people to access your information.

- Be careful with the use of colour on your PowerPoint slides, website material or documents. While colour adds impact, it can also make it difficult for some people to see. This might be because they have poor vision, or have colour blindness. About 8% of the population, mainly men, has some degree of inherited colour blindness, and as age increases colour vision has been found to deteriorate.[3] The most common problem is in distinguishing reds and greens. It is therefore sensible to avoid putting green text on a red background, or vice versa.
Other colour combinations can cause problems for some people. The best colour combinations are those with strong contrasts, either light text on a dark background, or dark text on a light background.
- Avoid the use of jargon. Every profession has its own language, which is fine if you only want others in your own profession to access your information. Heathcare, however, is a very interprofessional business and your information will most likely also be of interest to other professions, and to patients. Make sure that the language you use does not exclude them.
- If you are putting information on the Web, the World Wide Web Consortium (W3C) has design recommendations to make Web pages accessible. They offer 10 Quick Tips and additional guidance on their website. A search in any major search engine, such as Google, for 'W3C' and 'quick tips' will find this information, along with additional hints from a variety of sources.

References

1. Office of National Statistics, First Release, Internet Access, 2007. Available from www.statistics.gov.uk/hub/health-social-care/index.html [21 May 2009].
2. Australian Bureau of Statistics, *Household Use of Information Technology, Australia, 2006–07*. Report number 8146.0. Canberra: ABS, 2007. Available from www.abs.gov.au/AUSSTATS [21 May 2009].
3. Hertzberg R, Colour vision. *Aust N Z J Ophthalmol* 7 (3) 232–232. DOI :10.1111/j.1442-9071.1979.tb01429.x Available at www3.interscience.wiley.com/journal/119608449/abstract [8 August 2008].

4 Spreadsheets

Learning objectives

When this chapter is completed you will be able to:
- open, load and save spreadsheet files
- describe the cell process of data storage
- identify columns and rows of data
- understand and be able to work with worksheets
- carry out data manipulation and data presentation
- build a pivot table.

Extension material on pivot charts is available on the CD.

Generally, at the mention of spreadsheets all those with a maths aversion tend to move onto the next section – but if you do this, you will be missing out on a glorious application that really does save you time and energy and can make you look very skilled indeed. Although many people will use a spreadsheet rather like a database, using words, we shall be looking at the application as a superb aid to working with numbers.

As with all computer application software, it is vital that we make the software work for *us*, and not the other way round. In this chapter we shall examine the common uses for spreadsheets, and master these along with using spreadsheet data in other applications and presentations. The spreadsheet software we use in this book is Microsoft Excel, though many of the techniques are similar in other spreadsheet software.

4.1 The basics

To open a spreadsheet file, go to **Start** (bottom left of your screen), left-click, move the cursor over **All Programs** and find the icon in Figure 4.1, and left-click on it.

Figure 4.1 Excel icons for (left) Office 2007 and (right) Office 2003

When a spreadsheet file is opened, the very top (blue) line will state that it is Book 1 of Microsoft Excel, as shown in Figures 4.2 and 4.3.

Each time you open a new Excel file, you are actually opening a book (or workbook) of sheets, usually three at first opening. If you look towards the bottom of the Excel Window you will see tabs named Sheet1, Sheet2 and Sheet3. You can add more sheets if needed, but just for the moment let us accept that our Excel workbook is standard and contains three sheets (also called worksheets).

The orientation around any sheet, starting at the top, is much the same as for any application in the Microsoft Office suite, with a top menu line containing submenus and icons that you can hover over to get additional information or further submenus.

Many of the icons and menus on the main spreadsheet view will offer features with which you may be familiar from your use of Microsoft Word or Microsoft Access. For example: **New** for a new sheet; **Open** to access a previously saved sheet, **Save** to save the current sheet, etc. There will also be the format feature icons for text style, size, bold, centre and colours (to name but a few).

Additionally, there will be some new icons and menus, specific to Excel. We will cover all of these while looking at the basics.

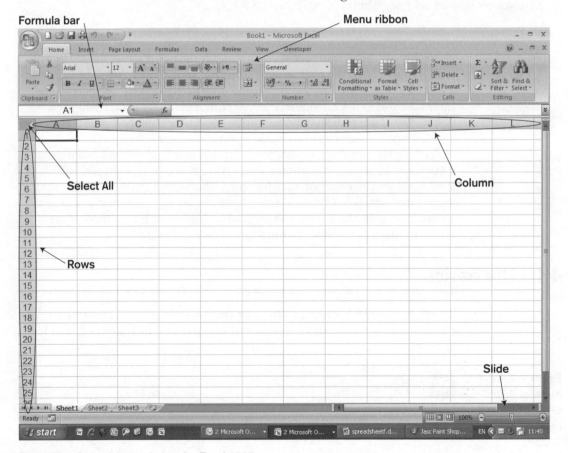

Figure 4.2 Spreadsheet window for Excel 2007

4.1.1   Columns, rows and cells

The main part of the screen is made up of boxes, called **cells**. These are referenced across the top in letters (commonly A to L are visible) – these are the **columns**. Down the left-hand side are numbers (commonly 1 to 33 are visible) – and these are called **rows**. Place your cursor (which will be a blocky cross shape) in the top-most, left-most cell, and left-click. You will see that just above the block of cells is a box containing the name A1; also the relevant cell is highlighted (a darker line around the outside of the cell), and the column letter and row number are coloured. If you now left-click on column G row 25, you will see that the highlight moves to G25 and the reference box states 'G25'. You can try as many of these clicks as you like; when you are ready, return to A1.

You can highlight (select) more than one cell at a time:

- To highlight a block of cells from C4 to H17, left-click and hold in cell C4 and then drag your mouse down and across to H17; then let go.
- To highlight an entire column, move your cursor over the letter of the column you are interested in, for example column C. The cursor will change to a down-arrow; left-click and you will see the column

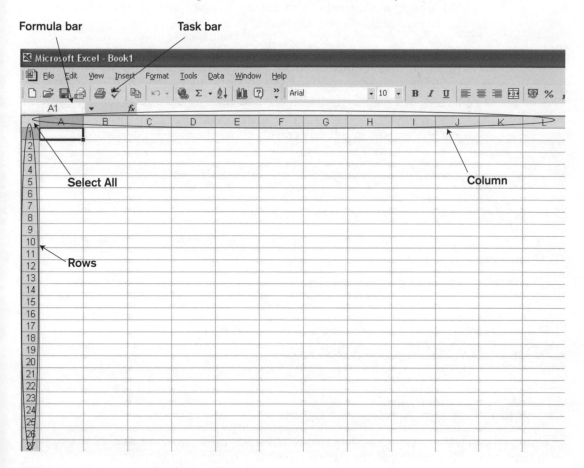

Figure 4.3 Spreadsheet window for Excel 2003

highlighted by a bold box and (commonly) a blue background. This column is now selected, and *everything* in the column will be included in whatever you do next – this can be dangerous, so use with caution. Left-click on any single cell to clear the column selection.

- To highlight a row, use exactly the same manoeuvre as for a column, but this time hover over one of the numbers down the left-hand side until you get a right-arrow, then left-click. Again, use this cautiously as everything in the row is now included in whatever you do next. Clear the same way as for columns.
- To highlight more than one entire column (or row), click in the first column letter box, hold and drag along the columns, then let go.

Each sheet is made up of thousands of cells, but for ease we are offered the initial window A1 to O33 (approximately). If you want to see the rest of the sheet, move your cursor to the bottom right of the Excel window where there are two slide bars, one horizontal and one vertical, and arrow buttons. On the horizontal line, press and hold the right arrow with your mouse pointer and you can get to column IV. On the vertical, press and hold the down arrow with your mouse pointer – and sit and wait until you get bored.

Go back to A1 when you are ready – a quick way to do this is to press CTRL-Up arrow on your keyboard.

Basic cell data entry

Each cell can only contain one piece of information. This information can be text, or a number, or a formula outcome. Each cell as shown initially is capable of varying in size, but we shall consider this later; for the moment, just concentrate on cell data entry.

EXERCISE 4.1

If you haven't already, open a new (blank) Excel workbook.

1   Move your cursor and highlight cell B4; this is now the 'active cell'. Enter the number 345.

2   Now highlight cell B5 – now the new 'active cell' – and enter the number 545.

3   Highlight cell B6, and enter the number 112.

We now want to do the sum 345 plus 545 multiplied by 112.

4   Highlight cell B7, and type in the formula:

   =(b4+b5)*b6

then press **Enter** (key ↵)
The formula will turn into the answer 99680.

Note that you can type in the cell references in lower-case (which is easier); the spreadsheet will automatically capitalise them for you.

We use the = character to inform the spreadsheet that we are about to key in a formula into a cell, to be calculated and the result displayed in that cell. Then, using basic mathematics, we add the two numbers together by placing them within brackets and adding the plus sign, then multiply (*) the result by the number in B6. (Note: to use the * sign, which represents multiplication in Excel, press SHIFT and number 8 together, written SHIFT+8. This is standard for UK, Australia, most of Europe and the USA.)

EXERCISE 4.1 CONTINUED

5 Try changing the number in B4 from 345 to 789. To do this, highlight the cell B4 and enter the number 789 – this overwrites the initial number. Then press the down arrow key (or right arrow key) to move away from the number you have just entered, and see what happens to the result.

You will see that the formula in B7 has remained the same, but has acknowledged that the number in B4 has changed and so has recalculated the result.
   In essence this is how all spreadsheets work, and maybe starts to show you just how helpful a spreadsheet could be in calculating results for you.

Basic auto-calculation

From Exercise 4.1 so far, you now have four numbers, all in column B, in rows 4, 5, 6 and 7 – but B7 is the result of a formula. We shall use these numbers to carry out some basic automatic calculations. Automatic calculations save us having to remember the formulae – but a word of caution: unless you have some very elementary knowledge of formulae, you will be placing all your trust in the program to do what you think it is doing. Blind faith is often a useful adjunct to one's armoury, and while we are in the realms of simple addition and the like there is no problem.

Excel provides a number of automatic calculations.

- In Excel 2007, go to the **Home** ribbon and look in the **Editing** section to find the sum sign Σ.
- In Excel 2003, look along the row of icons just below the top menu. Commonly, next to the Web link icon (a small globe with a chain link) is the sum sign Σ.

If you move your cursor over the icon, you will see it says 'AutoSum', and there is a list of further basic automatic calculations available by left-clicking the down-arrow next to the icon.

EXERCISE 4.1 CONTINUED

In order to operate any of the automatic functions available, we have to tell the program which numbers we wish to include in our calculation, so back to our B column.

6   Left-click on B4, thus highlighting the first figure 789, hold the mouse button down and drag the cursor downwards until all four numbers are included in the box, then let go. All four numbers should now be in a bold box, with the first in a white cell and the remainder in blue cells. If this doesn't happen first time have another go. If any of the numbers disappear don't worry, you can easily enter them in again.

7   Now move your cursor back up to the $\sum$ icon, click on the down-arrow to get to the submenu and then click on **Sum**.
    You should now have a fifth number in cell B8, which will be the result of adding up the first four numbers.

8   To check the calculation, left-click just in cell B8 and look up to the formula bar above your workbook. You will see the white box containing the cell reference B8, and to the right of this another, longer, white box labelled '*fx*' with the following formula in it:

$$=SUM(B4:B7)$$

Broken down into its component parts, this is:
❑   = SUM meaning *here comes a calculation and/or formula*, then
❑   (B4:B7) where the colon ':' indicates a list of cells from B4 to B7 inclusive. This is easier to state than B4+B5+B6+B7 but means the same thing.

Now we want to try a different calculation.

9   First delete the contents of B8 by highlighting it and pressing the **Delete** key.
    Now select cells B4 to B7 by left-clicking and dragging, then move to the $\sum$ icon and choose **Average** from the list in the down-arrow submenu. You will get a pretty big number because of B7, so you might like to try again without including B7 (just highlight B4 to B6 before going to the automatic calculation submenu).

10 Try out as many auto-calculations as you like, to get a feel for the sums being done.

When you are ready, we shall move on to Exercise 4.2.

Quick hint

A quick way to do AutoSum is to highlight the cell below the list of the items you want to add, then go to $\sum$ and choose **AutoSum**. A formula will appear in the highlighted cell; press the **Enter** key ($\leftarrow\!\!\!\rfloor$) and the result will appear.

One point to note: if there are cells in the column you are summing that have nothing in them, the auto-calculation will fail. In this case, you need to enter a zero into any empty cell before using AutoSum.

This works for most of the automatic calculations available.

Exercise 4.2

For this exercise, we shall be using pre-prepared data. This is held in a file called *Exercise 4-2.csv* which is available on the CD. If at any time you want to get a fresh copy from the CD, please do.

This file contains de-identified data, stored as comma-separated values, taken from a small group of students (nine in all, rows 3 to 11) who were using a virtual learning environment (VLE) for one of their modules during a course. Part of their marks came from joining in discussion forums, so the amount of time the students spent in the VLE and how often they visited the discussion forums was important information to gather.

1 To open the file, first open Excel. Then:
- ❏ In Excel 2007, go to **Office Button ➤ Open**
- ❏ In Excel 2003, go to **File ➤ Open.**

   Find the file *Exercise 4-2.csv*, left-click on it to select it and left-click on **Open**. Select where you want to save this file to – maybe in a folder just for use with this book, or a learning area on your computer drive; it is up to you. One point of warning: store files somewhere you can find then again, and create a back-up at least every week for your important files (see Chapter 2).
   Do a **Save As** and choose **Excel Workbook**.

2 You will notice that some of the text is not fully displayed in the columns. If you want to see the full text, left-click in the small grey box to the left of column A and above row 1 (this is the 'Select All' box). Your entire spreadsheet is now highlighted; next:
- ❏ in Excel 2007, go to **Home ➤ Cells ➤ Format ➤ AutoFit Column Width**
- ❏ in Excel 2003, go to **Format ➤ Column ➤ AutoFit Selection**.

You will see that the columns needing more width are now wider, and all the text is displayed. Click on a blank cell anywhere on your sheet to be ready for the next part of the exercise.

3 First, there are no totals for any of the columns. Working through each column, calculate the total for each column C to J.

4 Second, the averages of the student's time and discussions ('Read Messages' and 'Posted Messages') need to be calculated.

There are a couple of ways you could have attained the results to these two exercise questions: either by highlighting the column numbers and then going to AutoSum, or by clicking below each column in the first free cell and then going to AutoSum.

Both ways should have resulted in the following responses for step 3:

C	D	E	F	G	H	I	J
268	105:18:11	4685	98	52	60	716	803

If you did not get these results, then you need to re-examine how you carried out the calculation.

- One easy error to make is to miss cells with no data entered – you need to fill these in (with a zero in this instance) to ensure that all the rows in that particular column are included in the calculation. Look again, and see if there are any empty cells in the rows; if there are, enter a zero and recalculate.
- Another easy error to make is not highlighting all the numbers in the column; try again if you think this is the case.

Hopefully you noticed that the spreadsheet was able to do different calculations automatically. In column D the data are in time format – and the summing calculation has recognised this and converted the result into hours, minutes and seconds just as in the column data.

The results for part 4 should be:

D	E	F
11:42:01	520.5555556	10.88888889

This time, instead of 'Sum' you should have used 'Average'. Again, if you did not get these results please re-examine your calculation method.

In columns E and F we have a large number of decimal places (that is numbers after the decimal point). In most instances we only need two decimal places, and of course we can tell the sheet to present these two results to us to just two decimal places. First, highlight cells E12 and F12.

- In Excel 2007, now go to the **Home** ribbon; under the **Cells** section you will see **Format** and a down-arrow. Select **Format ➤ Format Cells** (Fig 4.4).

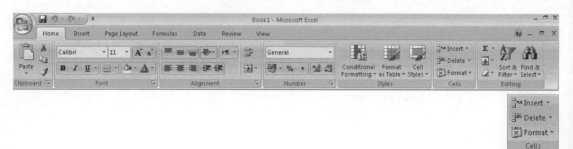

Figure 4.4 Format Cells area in Excel 2007

- In Excel 2003, now go to **Format ➤ Cell** and left-click. A sub-menu will appear (Fig 4.5):

Figure 4.5
Format Cells
dialog box

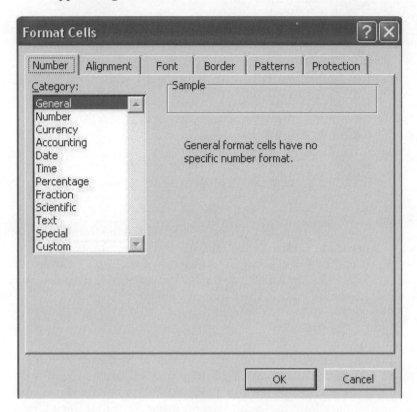

In the **Number** tab, click on 'Number', and you will be offered the opportunity to enter the number of decimal places you require. In this instance select '2' and left-click **OK**. Your number in E12 will now be displayed as 520.56, and in F12 the revised number will be 10.89.

We shall now try something a little more complicated before we complete this section.

EXERCISE 4.2 CONTINUED

5 Using a clean copy of *Exercise 4-2.csv* from the CD and saving it as an Excel workbook under a different filename, can you work out within the spreadsheet the average time each student spent using the virtual learning environment?

To complete part 5, you will use all the skills from the learning you have done above; however, you will also need a little bit of lateral thinking to complete the calculation.

The results you should get are:

3	00:29:51
4	00:03:49
5	00:24:23
6	00:16:38
7	00:31:47
8	00:28:10
9	00:18:27
10	00:38:15
11	00:11:59

For this part of the exercise, instead of moving from top to bottom, you needed to undertake the calculation *horizontally*, using the data in columns C and D. For ease you might have used column L in which to carry out your calculation; in which case for student number 1, their data is in row 3, and L3 should contain the following equation:

=(D3/C3)

that is, divide the information in cell D3 by the number in cell C3, then give the result. The answer is given in time format.

So that you do not have to key formulae in over and over, you can copy the formula down the column you are using. Type in the first formula (for row 3), and leave this cell highlighted. In the bottom right-hand corner of the cell is a little black box – grab this with your mouse (it will change to a + sign) and drag it down to row 11. The formula will 'fill down' the column, and will calculate correctly using the different data in each row. The same trick can be used to 'fill' a formula to the right across several rows – click and drag to the right. An alternative method is to type in the first formula, highlight that cell, and left-click and drag to include all the other cells you want the formula to appear in. The next step is:

- in Excel 2007, go to **Home ➤ Editing** and click on the blue down-arrow beneath the Σ sign
- in Excel 2003, go to **Edit ➤ Fill**

and choose **Down, Right** or another of the other options offered (Fig 4.6).

Figure 4.6 Filling options in Excel 2003

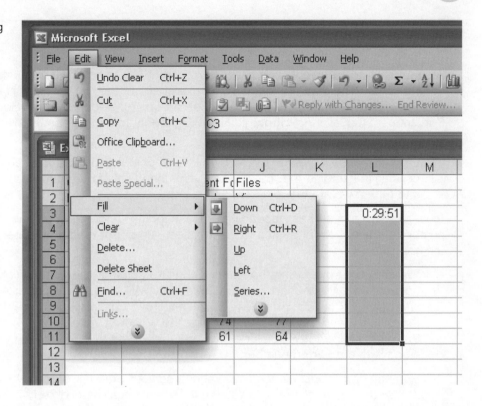

4.2 Sorting and filtering

Sorting and filtering data are very useful tools, particularly in a large spreadsheet.

4.2.1 Sorting spreadsheet data

Just as with any listing in a data collection, you can sort the data in a spreadsheet to meet your requirements. Some spreadsheet users actually prefer to use spreadsheets as a sort of database, but this works only for basic entries, such as a list of class members or house street numbers – in essence something fairly simple. We shall not be considering such use here, although an example of how this works is shown in the file *Conference Costing.xls* on the CD.

Exercise 4.3

A spreadsheet *Exercise 4-3.xls* is available on the CD to help you understand the sorting action. The data are taken from the website of the UK Office of National Statistics, and contains data on occupation groups for people living in South Yorkshire, at the levels of Strategic Health Authority (meaning county), region and country.

1   Open *Exercise 4-3.xls* in a new Excel workbook. If you want you can expand the cells as in Exercise 4.2, but it is really the long lists of numbers in columns E, F and G that we are interested in at this time.

Generally, we can sort as Ascending or Descending. Ascending puts the largest number at the bottom and rises to the smallest number at the top; Descending does the opposite.

2   We shall start by sorting the South Yorkshire column (E) to see which type of occupation is the most popular in the county. We need to include column A *and* column E in our sort – if we only highlighted column E, we would sort *only* this column, and it would then take ages to work out which occupation related to which number! If we include other columns, then this information will move along with our sorted numbers.

Remember that this is a long worksheet, so your drag will start at A1 and finish at E38 to include all the data you want. When it is all highlighted:
- ❐   in Excel 2007, go to **Home ➤ Editing ➤ Sort & Filter ➤ Custom Sort**
- ❐   in Excel 2003, go to **Data ➤ Sort**.

Figure 4.7
Editing section of Home ribbon, showing Sort & Filter

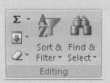

This opens a dialog box labelled **Sort**. Choose the column you want to sort on, which is E (it may already be offered as the main sort column). You will be asked whether you want Ascending (Smallest to Largest) or Descending (Largest to Smallest) order, and you may have the option of what type of data to sort on. Select descending order of values, and left-click on **OK**. The information will now be displayed in the sorted order. You can also just use the **Sort Ascending** and **Sort Descending** icons in the task bar in Excel 2003 (Fig 4.8).

Figure 4.8 Sort Ascending and **Sort Descending** icons in Excel 2003

Quick hint
In Excel 2007, if you want to sort by more than one column click on **Add Level** to add another row of options to sort by.

> **3** You may want to save your sorted file; choose an appropriate place to save it and give it a name such as *Exercise 4-3a.xls*.

4.2.2 Filtering spreadsheet data

Filter is a different technique to Sort. It does not re-arrange data; it is more like a sifting-out of things you want – and hiding items not required – i.e. acting like a search tool. It is generally used with large amounts (often called arrays) of data. There are two levels: AutoFilter and Advanced Filter.

EXERCISE 4.3 CONTINUED

4 Open a fresh copy of *Exercise 4-3.xls*, and select the block of cells E2 to G2.
  ☐ In Excel 2007, go to **Home ➤ Sort and Filter ➤ AutoFilter**.
  ☐ In Excel 2003, go to **Data ➤ Filter ➤ AutoFilter**.

Look at the sheet: you should now see small grey boxes with down-arrows to the right in columns E, F and G. These columns were selected for filtering as they contain the numeric data.

5 Left-click on the arrow on column E – this brings up the options shown in Figure 4.9 for Excel 2007, and those in Figure 4.10 for Excel 2003.

Figure 4.9
AutoFilter options in Excel 2007

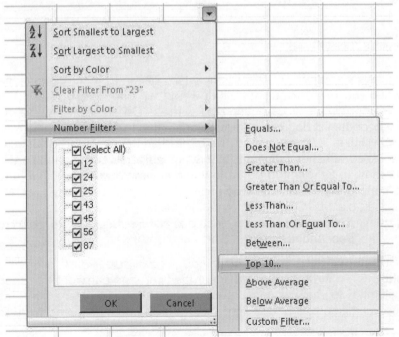

Figure 4.10
AutoFilter options
in Excel 2003

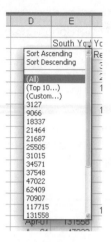

Excel 2007 has a few extra options to Excel 2003, for example Above Average, but if you select (Custom) in Excel 2003 you will be able to set up many of the extra options shown in Figure 4.9. The different options filter in different ways:

- (All) is pretty meaningless as it doesn't really change what you started with!
- Choosing (Top10 . . .) brings up a dialog box giving you three further options: Top or Bottom; how many; and Items or Percent.
- (Custom . . .) is pretty much the same as (Top10 . . .), except that you can do a lot more matching (searching) for things, including using more than one criteria.

EXERCISE 4.3 CONTINUED

6   Say we want the top 10% of our list in column E. In the options that come up when you left-click column E's down-arrow, choose (**Top10 . . .**), **then Top − 10 − Percent** in the three option boxes. Press **OK**. You will now be shown the top 10% of the list as filtered through column E.

You will know that it is column E that is being filtered because the arrow in the grey box turns blue, as do the relevant row and column numbers. The remainder of the sheet is still there – it is just hidden from view for this particular filter.

7   (Self-study) Using a clean copy of *Exercise 4-3.xls*, sort Column F into descending order.

8   (Self-study) Using another clean copy of *Exercise 4-3.xls*, filter column E to show the bottom 10%. Then clear the filter, and carry out a second filter using column E to show all items greater than 11465. To clear a filter, repeat the steps as if selecting for a filter, but 'turn off' the highlighted word **AutoFilter**.

Figure 4.11
Advanced Filter
options

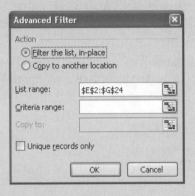

4.3 Formatting for clarity

Earlier, to save learning too many things all at once, we did some very rustic spreadsheet formatting. In this section we are going to carry out various aspects of formatting with considerably more finesse.

The more clearly viewable the spreadsheet, the more easily it can be read by you and others. If you are working with a spreadsheet you are probably pretty well versed in how it operates, but showing it to others may not be as easy as you think – especially when the other person is not so involved with the sheet as you are. Thus, formatting for your audience is vital in order to be as clear as possible with your presentation. Of course, some would argue that if you want to get something past a colleague without their full understanding you should make it as complicated as possible (*The Emperor's New Clothes* by Hans Christian Anderson, comes to mind). In this age of transparency such covert activity is uncalled-for and bad practice; indeed, should not be allowed – so clarity is what we are aiming for in this section.

4.3.1 Formatting a cell or group of cells

Sometimes the cell presented in the sheet does not display the whole of the information contained in that cell (or those cells) – it is cut off at the end. We need to expand the cells in order to help with clarity.

Earlier we just expanded the whole sheet: we highlighted the whole sheet and used:

- Home ➤ Cells ➤ Format ➤ AutoFit Column Width (Excel 2007)
- Format ➤ Columns ➤ AutoFit Selection (Excel 2003)

This added clarity but made our sheet very big to view on-screen; this time we shall try something a little different.

EXERCISE 4.4

1   Using a fresh copy of *Exercise 4-3.xls*, open the spreadsheet and save it under a suitable name, say *Exercise 4.4a-xls*. Highlight column A, then:
   ❒ in Excel 2007, go to **Home ➤ Cells ➤ Format ➤ Format Cells**
   ❒ in Excel 2003, go to **Format ➤ Cells**.

   Left-clicking on **Cells** will bring up a dialog box with tabs along the top; we are interested in **Alignment** (Fig 4.12). Go to **Text control** and select **Wrap text** then click on **OK**.

Figure 4.12
Format Cells
dialog box

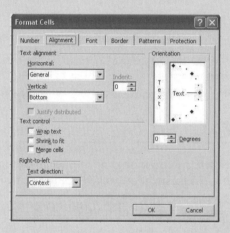

You will now be able to read all the text in the cells in column A. However, you will note that something else has happened: columns B, C and D are now empty; before, they were carrying the 'over' text. Also, you may find that the column that is now containing the wrapped text is *very* narrow.

2   For clarity, we don't want the now-empty columns B, C and D, so select them and:
   ❒ in Excel 2007, go to **Home ➤ Cells ➤ Delete**
   ❒ in Excel 2003, go to **Edit ➤ Delete**

   and left-click to remove these three columns. To widen column A, you're your cursor to the column A label at the top and hover over the right-hand vertical line until the cursor changes to a short line with two outward-pointing arrows. Click-and-drag to widen the column appropriately. (A similar technique can be used to change the depth of rows.)

Quick hint

Widening of columns is often used when doing calculations. If you see a row of ####### signs instead of the calculation result you expected, don't panic. It simply means the column is too narrow to show the number.

Note that the wrapping may have caused some disruption to full clarity. For example, select cell A6. The contents of this cell are displayed above the sheet in the *fx* part of the formula bar like this:

1. Managers and Senior Officials: 11. Corporate Managers

In other words, there are two pieces of information in A6. We can do one of two things: split the cell into two lines, or delete the first part as there is already a heading '1. Managers and Senior Officials' in A5.

3   Let us first split the one line into two. Go to the *fx* section, place your cursor just in front of the 11, and left-click. Then press **ALT+enter**; the result will be two lines of text (press **enter** again or move away from the active cell to see the final result).
    Sadly, there is no easy way to do this. You can of course set this two-line layout up at the outset of a new spreadsheet, which of course requires considerable forethought!

4   If we don't want to duplicate '1. Managers and Senior Officials', then again go in the *fx* section and this time delete '1. Managers and Senior Officials', leaving just '11. Corporate Managers'. Press **enter** or move away to see the result.

5   Things may not look as clear as you may want on screen, so it is a good idea to check with Print Preview:
    ❏   in Office 2007, go to **Office Button ➤ Print ➤ Print Preview**
    ❏   in Office 2003, go to **File ➤ Print Preview**.

    This will show you how your spreadsheet would appear on a page of A4 paper in portrait position. You can change page orientation, add or remove gridlines, show or hide column headings, and other things about the way your spreadsheet looks by left-clicking on **Setup** in the menu available in Print Preview. (Fig 4.13)
    Left-click on **Close** in Print Preview to move back to the spreadsheet.

Figure 4.13
Page Setup
options for
printing a
spreadsheet

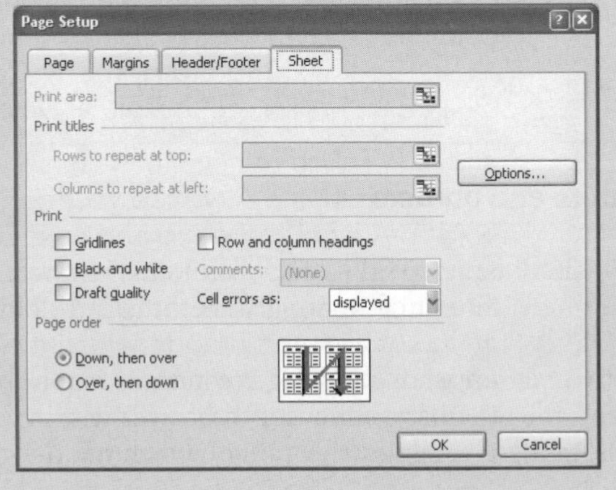

4.3.2 Formatting a column heading

There is another way we can format cells, which is particularly helpful for column titles.

---

*EXERCISE **4.4** CONTINUED*

6 We shall use the same Cell Alignment tool as in the first part of this exercise. This time, highlight:
- ❐ either B2 to D3 if you are using a fresh copy of *Exercise 4-3.xls*
- ❐ or E2 to G3 if you done and saved the steps above.

Now:
- ❐ in Excel 2007, go to **Home ➤ Cells ➤ Format ➤ Format Cells**
- ❐ in Excel 2003, go to **Format ➤ Cells**
to bring up the Format Cells dialog box (Fig 4.12).

Under the tab **Alignment** you should see **Orientation** and a semi-circle with a horizontal line; this shows the current alignment of the text in these highlighted cells. Grab the red diamond with your mouse and drag the horizontal line upwards to the vertical position. Let go and press **OK**. Your text will now be aligned vertically. Preview your spreadsheet.

Sadly, in Print Preview the results of question 6 don't look too good. Another solution is to combine the heading text for one column into one cell instead of two.

7 Use the *fx* (insert function) box and the **ALT+enter** command to type or copy the text from row 3 into the relevant cells in row 2. We now need to hide row 3. Highlight this row and:
- ❐ in Excel 2007, go to **Home ➤ Cells ➤ Format ➤ Visibility ➤ Hide & Unhide ➤ Hide Rows**
- ❐ in Excel 2003, go to **Format ➤ Row ➤ Hide**.

Print Preview your spreadsheet – things should be gradually looking better and clearer.

8 When you are happy with your formatting, don't forget to save your sheet.

4.3.3 Formatting using colours and borders

Less is more – don't be tempted to overdo colours; but note that at times, and if used in moderation, highlighting something in colour can help with clarity.

There are two main reasons for using colour: one is for presentation formatting, and the other is to show key indicators within a spreadsheet (such as a loss, gain, or result outside range) which might otherwise be missed.

EXERCISE 4.4 CONTINUED

9 Using a new copy of *Exercise 4-3.xls*, open the sheet and highlight E2 to G3. Then:
   ❏ in Excel 2007, go to **Home ➤ Cells ➤ Format ➤ Format Cells**
   ❏ in Excel 2003, go to **Format ➤ Cells**.

   Using **Fill** (Excel 2007) or the **Patterns** tab (Excel 2003), select a colour and left-click **OK**. You can see your results in Print Preview.

10 For a border, use the same technique as in question 9, but this time use the **Borders** tab. Select an outline around the cell(s). Preview your spreadsheet.

4.3.4 Formatting using preset template(s)

Quick hint

Note that right-clicking on the Sheet1 tab gives you access to a whole range of options to do with sheets, including inserting new sheets and renaming them. Be careful when using Delete, though, as you cannot undo the deletion of a sheet!

As with all applications within the Microsoft Office suite, there is an opportunity to start your sheet with a preset format – a template. These are limited, but do give you an idea of what can be achieved.

To use a template, open a new, empty spreadsheet and right-click the **Sheet1** tab at the bottom left of the sheet. Choose **Insert ➤ Spreadsheet Solutions**.

You will be offered a choice of available templates; click on any of these to view.

Exercise 4.5 below will test your skills learnt from section 4.3. As you are free to do almost anything to improve the clarity of the supplied workbook, it is impossible to give an 'answer' – but you will know whether you have succeeded or not!

EXERCISE 4.5

Using the *Exercise 4-5.xls* spreadsheet provided, prepare the sheet for discussion with another colleague in a clear and easily understood manner.

4.4 Analysis and statistical tools

So far, we have done much of the work required to build our spreadsheet; now it is time to get some just rewards from our learning. We are now going to get the sheet data and application software to work for us in analysing data.

Indeed, we have already done a number of mathematical functions with our different spreadsheets: we have counted the number of items in a column; worked out the top and/or bottom 10% of a list of numbers; worked out the average of a list of numbers, and found the total or sum of a list of numbers. Here we shall look at bit more at percentages, carry out a count and some other basic maths, and then get into the realms of statistics.

4.4.1   Non-statistical calculation and manipulation

Percentage

You may want to use a simple percentage calculation, to show the number of occurences per 100. For example, 5 occurences out of 25 cases = 20%. You might use such calculations to assess what would happen if something, for example the cost of a required product, was to increase (or decrease) by different percentages. Later, in the section on pivot tables, we shall look at more complex percentage calculations.

EXERCISE 4.6

1   Open a new, blank spreadsheet. Then:
   ❑ in cell C4, enter the number 454 representing the cost of an item
   ❑ in cell D4, enter 4%
   ❑ in cell E4, enter the formula =c4*(1+d4)
   and press **Enter**.

   The result in cell E4 will be 454 plus 4% = 472.16. Try changing the amount in D4 (either lower or higher) to see the outcome.

2   You have probably guessed the next bit: removing a given per cent from a figure. To do this:
   ❑ in cell C6 enter 454 again, and in D6 enter 4%
   ❑ in cell E6, enter the formula =c6*(1-d6)
   and press **Enter**.

   The result in cell E6 will be 454 minus 4% = 435.84. Again, you can change D6 to see alternative outcomes dependent upon the percentage being used.

What-if?

One of the glories of spreadsheets is that they allow us to carry out mathematical assessment of potential or actual change. This might be the opening or closing of a care unit; employing more staff or increasing temporary staff (or vice versa). On a personal level, this could involve looking at changing our income and expenditure to afford a much-wanted vacation. Change almost always includes a cost (i.e. numbers), so what better tool to use than a spreadsheet to look at the outcome of the change?

EXERCISE 4.7

Imagine that your manager has agreed on the allocation of an additional 30,000 (use your own monetary unit) over the next six months and seeks your views on how best to use this for your clinical unit. You know that the best solution would be hiring another member of staff, but you are aware that employing staff entails an additional cost to the published salary, so-called 'employer costs'. These employer costs account for an additional 25% for a full-time member of staff, 20% for part-timers who work between 50% and 90%, and 15% for a staff member under 50% of the time. The basic salary for the grade and level of staff member you want is 42,000 per annum.

1   Using a new spreadsheet and appropriate explanatory headings, enter:
    ❏   42,000 into cell B2 – the published salary figure
    ❏   100% into cell C2 – the percentage of a full-time position
    ❏   25% into cell D2 – the maximum employer costs
    ❏   =b2*c2(1+d2) into cell E2 – to calculate total costs (published salary plus employer cost)
    ❏   =e2/2 into cell E2 – the calculation for half a year.

The outcome for a 50% part-time staff member will be 26,250, which is inside your allocation. However, your manager informs you that there are further costs associated with advertising and application processes amounting to 3,250, and the Supplies department has sent you a message stating that their costs to your clinical unit will increase by 5% over the next six months; over the last six months you spent a total of 86,554, and any extra will need to come out of the 30,000. How do these affect your plans?

2   We can work out the effect of the further costs in cell G2 using the formula:

    =f2+3250

    We can type in the actual figure of 3250 as this is a static figure.
    The further costs don't affect your plans, but do push it very close to the limit.

3   Now to deal with the Supplies account. What would 5% add to 86,554?
    ❏   In cell A8 enter a heading 'Supplies' (and use this rest of this row for explanatory headings).
    ❏   In cell B9 enter the known figure of 86,554 – cost over last six months.
    ❏   In cell C9 enter 5% – the amount the Supplies costs will rise by.
    ❏   In cell D9 enter the formula =b9*c9 – the amount of the increase.

Oops! It appears as though our additional Supplies costs are going to take us over the extra amount on offer, so we need to go back to our new employee costs and try some different scenarios.

4   Copy cells B2 to H2 down two or three rows and try some 'what if' scenarios using the data provided at the beginning of this exercise. For example:
   ❏ a 50% part-timer for six months
   ❏ a 75% part-timer for six months.

Try some other percentages to see how you can get the maximum value from the 30,000 in terms of extra employee time.

Count and other useful calculations

One area where a spreadsheet is ideal is to help with the planning of a conference; there is much we can do to save effort if the spreadsheet is set up correctly. In the worked example below, which works through some useful spreadsheet functions, we will use more than one worksheet to help us with our calculations, as otherwise things get very confusing.

Worked example 4.8

A simulated conference costing spreadsheet, *Conference Costing.xls*, has been provided on the CD. Please note that this is purely to demonstrate some additional features of a spreadsheet, and should not be used as a template for costing a real conference.
   Open the spreadsheet, and use it to work through the following text.

On the first sheet of *Conference Costing.xls* there is very little information, but have a look towards the bottom of the screen. You will see that the three sheets have been named 'Master', 'Calculations' and 'Delegates'. Click on each sheet to see what they contain.
   The idea here is to have the main bulk of information and calculations hidden from view, so that if you want a quick look at the current state of play you are not searching around what would probably be a far more complicated screen to find important information.

We will now look more closely at the **Delegates** sheet. The basic information here, as you would expect, is about the delegates. This sheet can be used to carry out a Mail Merge in Microsoft Word (see Chapter 3, section 3.1.6) to create delegate lists, delegate labels/badges and anything else where we want delegate names. An example of merged delegate badges can be found in the file *Delegate Badges1.doc*.
   There are some vital operations in the **Delegates** sheet which are then used elsewhere in the other sheets in this workbook.

a COUNTA

This is used in cell G7, and demonstrates how the number of cells with text can be counted. COUNTA is a very simple calculation; all it does is count the number of filled cells in a given range. Here the range is A3 to A100, which allows for additional delegates as time progresses towards the conference date. G7 contains the formula:

=COUNTA(A3:A100)

b COUNTIF

Used in cells G13 and G16. This function is also used with text cells, this time in the range E3 to E100.

- In cell G13, we only want to count those cells that have the word 'Full' in them. G13 gives the formula:

=COUNTIF(E3:E100,"Full")

This means that within our chosen range (E3 to E100), only those cells containing the word 'Full' will be counted. Note the use of double quote marks – these indicate that the text to be counted must be exactly, and only, the word 'Full'.

In G16 we have used COUNTIF again, but this time to show only 'Day' delegates by using the formula:

=COUNTIF(E3:E100,"Day")

c SUM

In cell G10 the operation of SUM has been used to add all the numbers in the range D3 to D100.

d Copying cells into different sheets in the same workbook

Each sheet has its own reference label, so a cell on the Delegates sheet is really:

Delegates!D3

While we are working *within* the Delegates sheet, we don't have to include the sheet reference. Note the use of '!' – this is a bit like the '➤' we have been using to say 'next part'.

If we now open the Calculations sheet and highlight D3, you will see the operation command:

=Delegates!G7

This instructs the spreadsheet to copy the data from cell G7 in the Delegates sheet to this cell here, in the Calculations sheet. Similarly, I3 copies data from cell G10 in the Delegates sheet.

What-if? using pivot tables

Pivot tables frighten most people, probably because the name sounds imposing but not in any way obvious. They can also look complicated. Forget the name – the technique is a useful one, and once you've worked through creating one you will see how surprisingly easy this is to do.

We'll walk through the process in Exercise 4.8, doing some of the same reports as in the previous sections but using pivot tables instead. Then we'll show some uses which are much easier done with pivot tables than with simple formulae.

Worked example 4.9

There is an expanded version of the simulated conference costing spreadsheet on the CD, called *Conference Pivot.xls*. Open the spreadsheet and familiarise yourself with it. We will use it in Exercise 4.9.

You will see that it is very similar to the previous workbook, with a few changes and some additional columns of data. As for the previous workbook, please note that this is just to demonstrate some features of spreadsheets and should not be used as a template for managing a real conference.

The changes in *Conference Pivot.xls* are on the Delegates sheet. First, the blank line underneath the column titles in the previous workbook (Surname, First Name, Title and so on) has been removed. This makes life easier because it lets Excel work out where the data table starts and ends, and allows it to recognise the column titles as names for the information in each column.

Second, we have added some more columns, to the right of the column called 'Type' in the previous spreadsheet. These add information to each row of the table, and make it look a little bit more like an extract from a database.

Think of each column in the Delegates sheet of *Conference Pivot.xls* as the name of a piece of data, which each row possesses: so each row has a Surname, a First Name, a Type, a Diet, and so on.

Using the Pivot Table feature, we can perform some quick rearrangements of this table. Nearly all useful rearrangements will take just a small number of the columns and use their contents to populate a new table, a pivot table in fact.

EXERCISE 4.9

1   First, we will do a count of 'Full' entries, but this time using a pivot table. Position your mouse somewhere within the table on the **Delegates** sheet (if this confuses you, then let's say click on 'Scotland', about half-way down). Then:
  ❏ in Excel 2007, go to **Insert ➤ PivotTable**
  ❏ in Excel 2003, go to **Data ➤ PivotTable and PivotChart Report.**

Figure 4.14
Accessing the pivot table function in (left) Excel 2007 and (right) Excel 2003

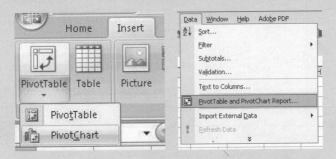

Pivot tables are handled quite differently in Excel 2007 and Excel 2003, so we will deal with each separately. Skip whichever section does not apply to you.

2   **Excel 2007**
    Choosing **PivotTable** brings up the dialog box shown in Figure 4.15.

Figure 4.15
Create Pivot Table dialog box in Excel 2007

Excel has spotted the table to use, because we formatted it in a way it likes (by putting in column titles and leaving out blank formatting lines). If you look at your spreadsheet data beneath the Create Pivot Table dialog box, you will see that the table is selected – a flickering dashed line is shown around the cells to be included in the pivot table. Left-click on **OK**.

A new sheet opens, with the outline of a pivot table on the left and a panel containing the names of our columns on the right (Fig 4.16). This is where we choose what columns of information should be used to produce the pivot table. Here we're going to use just the 'Type' column, because that's all we are interested in at the moment.

Figure 4.16
Outline pivot table in Excel 2007

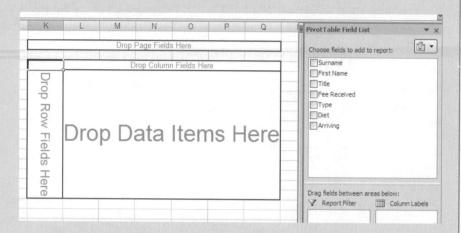

Left-click on **Type** in the right-hand panel, and drag it over to where it says 'Drop Column Fields Here'. You should see 'Type' appearing in row 3, with 'Data', 'Full' and 'Grand Total' beneath. Now drag **Type** into the 'Drop Data Fields Here' area as well, and see that the words 'Count of Type' appear in cell A3 (Fig 4.17).

Figure 4.17
Pivot table based on the 'Type' column, in Excel 2007

	A	B	C	D
1	Drop Page Fields Here			
2				
3	Count of Type	Type ▼		
4		Day	Full	Grand Total
5	Total	2	23	25

You can look in the **Options** ribbon in Excel 2007 to see all the functions within a pivot table that you can change (Fig 4.18).

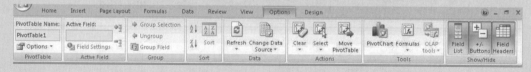

Figure 4.18 Options ribbon in Excel 2007, showing pivot table functions

The final section **Show/Hide** is where layout can be adjusted in Excel 2007.

3 Excel 2003
Excel 2003 starts up a three-step Wizard (Fig 4.19).

Figure 4.19
Step 1 of Pivot
Table Wizard in
Excel 2003

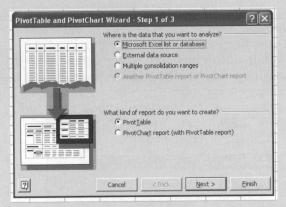

In Step 1, accept the defaults, which tell Excel that the data are in Excel and that we wish to create a table, not a table and a chart. Left-click **Next** for Step 2 (Fig 4.20).

Figure 4.20
Step 2 of Pivot
Table Wizard in
Excel 2003

Excel has spotted the table to use, because we formatted it in a way it likes (by putting in column titles and leaving out blank formatting lines). If you look at your spreadsheet data beneath the Wizard box, you will see that the table is selected – a flickering dashed line is shown around the cells to be included in the pivot table. Left-click **Next** to move to Step 3 (Fig 4.21).

Figure 4.21
Step 3 of Pivot
Table Wizard in
Excel 2003

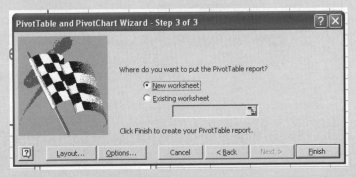

This allows you to chose where to put the resulting pivot table. The default puts it into a new worksheet, which is fine by us. It also cunningly conceals the real guts of this Wizard behind the **Layout** button. Do *not* choose Finish; instead, left-click on **Layout**.

This is where we choose what columns of information should be used to produce the pivot table. Here we're going to use just the 'Type' column, because that's all we are interested in at the moment.

Left-click on the **Type** button on the right, and drag it over to the word 'COLUMN' in the mock-up picture of the table, in the middle of the window. You should see 'Type' appearing in the top of the picture. Now drag **Type** into the 'DATA' area as well, and see that the words 'Count of Type' appear in the middle of the picture (Fig 4.22).

Figure 4.22
Placing fields into a pivot table in Excel 2003

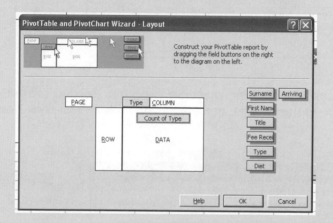

Finally, press **OK**. This takes you back to the previous dialog box, and you can now press **Finish**. Figure 4.23 shows the pivot table along with the Pivot Table toolbar, where you can adjust the layout in Excel 2003.

The result will be a new pivot table, in a new worksheet, looking like this:

Figure 4.23
Pivot table based on the 'Type' column, in Excel 2003, showing Pivot Table toolbar

	A	B	C	D	E	F
1						
2						
3	Count of Type	Type ▼				
4		Day	Full	Grand Total		
5	Total	2	23	25		
6						
7		PivotTable			▼ ✕	
8		PivotTable ▼				
9						
10						

The result in Excel 2007 is very similar:

Figure 4.24
Pivot table based on the 'Type' column, in Excel 2007

	A	B	C	D
1		Drop Page Fields Here		
2				
3	Count of Type	Type ▼		
4		Day	Full	Grand Total
5	Total	2	23	25

From Figures 4.23 and 4.24 we can see that there are two rows with 'Day' in the 'Type' column, and 23 rows with 'Full' in the same column. Or in other words, we have done much the same as using the =COUNTIF formula in the previous workbook.

A couple of points to note about this:

1 We based the new pivot table on the 'Type' column only – no rows. We will show an example with a row later on, but this is about the simplest pivot table that makes any sense.

2 We used the same column (the 'Type' column) as the data – this is a shorthand way of telling Excel that we want to count the values rather than do any arithmetic on them.

---

*EXERCISE **4.9** CONTINUED*

4 Now create a new pivot table within the Delegates sheet of *Conference Pivot.xls* using the same procedure as above – the only difference is going to be which columns and rows you set up for the new table.

You will probably get a message along these lines (Fig 4.25):

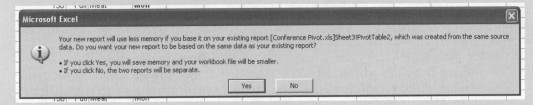

Microsoft Excel

Your new report will use less memory if you base it on your existing report [Conference Pivot.xls]Sheet3!PivotTable2, which was created from the same source data. Do you want your new report to be based on the same data as your existing report?

• If you click Yes, you will save memory and your workbook file will be smaller.
• If you click No, the two reports will be separate.

[Yes]   [No]

Figure 4.25 Using the same source data for a new pivot table

You can answer Yes or No here, as the fancy takes you, although answering **Yes** is probably the most useful response.

In Excel 2003, when you get to the final dialog box, don't forget to press the **Layout** button.

Set out your pivot table layout as shown in Figure 4.26.

Figure 4.26 Layout for a more complicated pivot table

PivotTable and PivotChart Wizard - Layout

Construct your PivotTable report by dragging the field buttons on the right to the diagram on the left.

PAGE   Type   COLUMN   Surname   Arriving
       Fee Rece   First Nam
                   Count of Type   Title
       ROW   DATA   Fee Rece
                                             Type
                                             Diet

[Help]   [OK]   [Cancel]

As well as dragging 'Type' over to the column and data areas, we have also dragged 'Fee Received' to the row part of the pivot table layout.

The result should be similar to before, with the difference that we now have a few more rows in the new table (Fig 4.27):

Figure 4.27
More complicated pivot table example

	A	B	C	D
1				
2				
3	Count of Type	Type ▼		
4	Fee Received ▼	Day	Full	Grand Total
5	0		1	1
6	100	2		2
7	150		22	22
8	Grand Total	2	23	25

From this, we can do a quick check that the Day attendees have paid the reduced rate, and the Full attendees have paid the full rate – and also see that one attendee has paid nothing at all.

Next we will explore *why* these are called pivot tables (part of the reason is that previous spreadsheet packages had used other names, but there is more to it than that).

5 In the pivot table you got as a result of question 4, try dragging the 'Fee Received' button to where the 'Type' one is, and then dragging the 'Type' one to where the 'Fee Received' one used to be. In other words, swap the column names with the rows name. You will have *pivoted* the table. See Figure 4.28.

Figure 4.28
Pivoting a pivot table

	A	B	C	D	E
1			Drop Page Fields Here		
2					
3	Count of Type	Fee Received ▼			
4	Type ▼	0	100	150	Grand Total
5	Day		2		2
6	Full	1		22	23
7	Grand Total	1	2	22	25

This way round may be more useful to you, depending on what you want the pivot table report for – it often pays to 'play' with a table like this to see what shows your data most clearly.

There are more things you can do with a pivot table, but here are the essential points:

- Pivot tables are based on data tables, usually stored in the same spreadsheet although they may be stored elsewhere.
- Pivot tables are nearly always a summary or extract of existing data, reorganised to pick out certain information that is not readily apparent in the original form.

- Most of the time, the pivot table will have columns with names taken from the data of the original table (e.g. 'Full' and 'Day' in our example were not columns in the original table, but data values in the 'Type' column).

EXERCISE 4.10 (SELF-STUDY)

You might like to experiment with pivot tables a bit more. Using a fresh copy of *Conference Pivot.xls*, see if you can produce a result like this:

	A	B	C	D	E	F
1						
2						
3	Count of Arriving	Arriving ▼				
4	Diet ▼	Mon	Tue	Wed	Sun	Grand Total
5	Gluten Free	2				2
6	Halal	2				2
7	Meat	11	2	1	3	17
8	Vegan	1				1
9	Vegetarian	3				3
10	Grand Total	19	2	1	3	25

4.4.2 Statistical calculation and manipulation

In any spreadsheet there will be opportunity to undertake a number of statistical functions on your data; Excel is no different.

The statistical tools are not necessarily installed automatically when you install the Office suite, but they can be added easily without additional cost. First, check to see if they *are* already installed or not.

In Excel 2007:

- Go to **Office Button ➤ Excel Options**. Choose **Add-Ins**, and look near the top to see if **Analysis ToolPak** is an active application Add-In.
- If not, go to **Manage** (at the bottom of the screen), ensure **Excel Add-Ins** is selected, and press **Go**.
- In the **Add-Ins available** box, select the **Analysis ToolPak** check box, and then click **OK**.
- If you get prompted that the Analysis ToolPak is not currently installed on your computer, press **Yes** to install it.

In Excel 2003:

- Go to **Tools** and look at the submenu to see if there is an option that says **Data Analysis,** often near the bottom of the drop-down list (you will probably need to click on the double down-arrows).
- If not, go to **Tools ➤ Add-Ins**. In the list of **Add-Ins available**, put a check mark in the box next to **Analysis ToolPak** and then press **OK**.
- If you get prompted that the Analysis ToolPak is not currently installed on your computer, press **Yes** to install it.

> **Quick hint**
> If **Analysis ToolPak** is not listed in the **Add-Ins available** box, click **Browse** to locate it.

After you have loaded the Analysis ToolPak:

- in Excel 2007, the **Data Analysis** command is available in the **Analysis** ribbon on the **Data** tab
- in Excel 2003, go to **Tools ➤ Data Analysis** (which is now visible).

You will get a dialog box (Fig 4.29) containing the preset statistical tests available for you to carry out on data. We shall look at three to give you a flavour of how things work; as your needs grow, you can explore further ones. The three we shall examine are: Descriptive Statistics, Histogram and t-test: Paired Two Sample for Means.

Figure 4.29 Data Analysis options

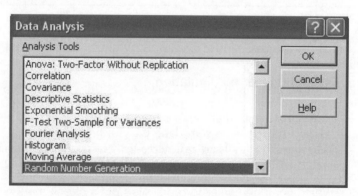

Descriptive Statistics

This is the first stage of analysis, where you get a lot of information at a basic level, and it is a good introduction to statistical tools.

EXERCISE 4.11

1 Open the file *Demographic and health indicators.xls* provided on the CD. This is a large file, and we shall be using sections of the data for our analysis.

2 Open the **Data Analysis** dialog box (see above for how) and select **Descriptive Statistics** from the available items. You will get a further dialog box, as shown in Figure 4.30.

Figure 4.30
Options in
Descriptive
Statistics

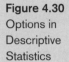

You will first be asked for a range of data to which the Descriptive Statistics will apply; the Input Range. This must be two or more columns or rows (usually columns). Check that your cursor is blinking in the empty Input Range in the empty box; you can now select your range.

3 For demonstration purposes, click and drag to select C19 to D29 – thus including two columns. When you release the mouse, this range should show up in the **Input Range** box. Under **Grouped by** check that **Columns** is selected (rather than Rows).

4 Next are the Output options. It is generally safer at this stage to have the result presented in a new sheet, so check that **New worksheet ply** is selected, and in its white box type a sensible name that will have meaning for you, for example *descriptive stats C19:D29*. If you want to place your result in a new workbook (a new spreadsheet) you can, but here we will keep it fairly simple.

5 Put a check mark next to **Summary statistics** – this will show one statistic on one line, which is much easier to read. Also put a check mark next to **Confidence Level for Mean**, usually set at 95%.

The confidence level is a measure of how confident you are that the sample size is adequate for the results given. Having it set to 95% means that you are 95% certain that the sample size is okay. If set at 99%, this would suggest almost total confidence in the sample size; so to allow for a little flexibility, 95% is acceptable.

6 The **Kth Largest** and **Kth Smallest** are already set to 1; these give you the largest and smallest number in the data columns. You can put your own number in these categories, but again for ease we shall leave them as 1.

7 When you are ready, press **OK**. You will be presented, on a new sheet, with a set of results like those in Figure 4.31 (you may need to AutoFit or widen the columns to see everything.)

Column1		Column2	
Mean	715.85	Mean	626.8
Standard Error	12.6337	Standard Error	10.85142
Median	719.25	Median	624
Mode	#N/A	Mode	#N/A
Standard Deviation	39.95128	Standard Deviation	34.31521
Sample Variance	1596.105	Sample Variance	1177.533
Kurtosis	-0.13294	Kurtosis	-1.35842
Skewness	0.510488	Skewness	0.133929
Range	123.5	Range	98.1
Minimum	668.8	Minimum	582.7
Maximum	792.3	Maximum	680.8
Sum	7158.5	Sum	6268
Count	10	Count	10
Confidence Level (95.0%)	28.57945	Confidence Level (95.0%)	24.54764

Figure 4.31 Results of Descriptive Statistics function

Table 4.1 explains what each of these results means.

Table 4.1 Explanation of components of Descriptive Statistics

Mean	Measures the average of a set of data (sometimes called 'arithmetic mean').
Standard Error	Measures the reliability of the data used; the higher the number, the more reliable.
Median	Measures the central point over a number of values; it is different to the mean in that it is a true central point, not an arithmetic calculation.
Mode	Gives you the most frequently occurring number in a data set. Ours has come back as #N/A meaning 'not available', suggesting that there are no duplicate numbers in either column examined.
Standard Deviation	This measures the dispersion of a sample or, put another way, the amount of variation from the mean in a single sample of data. It is expressed in points: the higher the number, the wider (worse) the dispersion.
Sample Variance	Another measure of dispersion.

(Table 4.1 continued)

Kurtosis	In a frequency distribution curve with peaks (a bell curve), kurtosis measures the pointedness of the peak and the length of the 'tails' at either end of the curve. A positive kurtosis number indicates that the curve is more peaked than a normal distribution curve; there is a higher probability that values are close to the mean. A negative kurtosis number indicates that the curve is flatter compared with a normal distribution curve; values are spread more widely between the mean and the extreme values.
Skewness	This is a measurement of the degree of asymmetry in a distribution. If skewness is negative, the data are spread out more to the left of the mode than to the right. If skewness is positive, the data are spread out more to the right of the mode. The skewness of any symmetric distribution is zero.
Range	This is the length of the smallest interval which contains all the data. It is calculated by subtracting the smallest observations from the greatest, and provides an indication of statistical dispersion.
Minimum	The lowest number in the series of data.
Maximum	The highest number in the series of data.
Sum	The total of the series of data added together.
Count	The number of data items in the series.
Confidence Level 95%	The measure of the degree of confidence you can have in the results of your analysis; the nearer to zero, the better the confidence.

You can see that there is a lot of useful information on the data supplied.

8 (Self-study) Feel free to try out this Descriptive Statistics test on other data held within this spreadsheet at your leisure.

Histogram

In data analysis, the histogram is one of the tools that determines the quality of the data and the results being presented. A histogram may look like a normal bar chart, but it is not. We shall now examine the complex way in which a histogram actually presents its results.

A histogram is a graphical display of frequencies from the data. Not only are we dealing with the numbers as we see them before us in our spreadsheet, we are measuring the *frequency intervals* between that data in the spreadsheet – that is what a histogram does. A histogram is a type of bar graph that uses the width of the bars to represent the various classes (e.g. marks awarded), and the height of the bars to represent their relative frequencies (e.g. number of times the class [marks] can be said to occur).

EXERCISE 4.12

1   Open a clean copy of *Demographic and health indicators.xls*, bring up the list of functions under **Data Analysis**, and select **Histogram**.

2   Click and drag to enter the data range E19 to E29. Don't enter anything in the 'Bin' box – if this is blank, the spreadsheet will assume that the intervals are evenly spread.

3   Select **New worksheet ply** and give it a sensible name, then select **Chart Output** (leave the other boxes blank), and press **OK**.

You will be presented with two things: a table and a chart – see Figure 4.32.

Figure 4.32
Results of the
Histogram
function

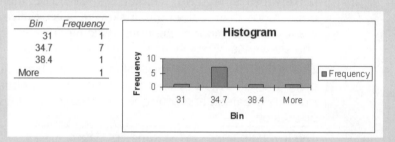

So, we are presented with a graph that uses the width of the bars to represent the various classes (31 to more than 38.4), and the height of the bars to represent their relative frequencies.

4   (Self-study) Feel free to practise on other sections of the main spreadsheet to see how you fare with histograms.

t-test: Paired Two Sample for Means

A t-test is a common parametric statistical test of the difference between the means of two data samples. 'Parametric' means a type of statistical test that assumes a normal distribution in the data. Non-parametric statistical tests are used when data cannot be meaningfully added or subtracted; they are less sensitive than parametric tests, but can be useful on very large collections of data.

EXERCISE 4.13

1   Open a clean copy of *Demographic and health indicators.xls* and open the list of Data Analysis functions available. Select **t-Test: Paired Two Sample for Means** and click on **OK**.

2 The sections of data we shall take are L20 to L29, and M20 to M29. Note that the two data ranges you are comparing must contain the same number of data items. Use click and drag to enter L20 to L29 in the 'Variable 1 Range' box, and to enter M20 to M29 in the 'Variable 2 Range' box.

3 We are dealing here with age ranges, so we are going have a hypothesis range of zero – indicating that our hypothesis is that the means of the two ranges. Type a zero in the 'Hypothesized Mean Difference' box.

4 The 'Alpha' range is a value from zero to 1, indicating the confidence level. Commonly 0.05 is used, which suggests that our confidence level is 95% for the test.

5 Select **New worksheet ply** and give it a suitable name, for example *t-test*, and press **OK**.

The results will look something like Figure 4.33; the different elements are explained in Table 4.2.

t-Test: Paired Two Sample for Means		
	Variable 1	*Variable 2*
Mean	74.58889	79.6
Variance	4.741111	2.4425
Observations	9	9
Pearson Correlation	0.999129	
Hypothesized Mean Difference	0	
df	8	
t Stat	-24.2722	
P(T<=t) one-tail	4.43E-09	
t Critical one-tail	1.859548	
P(T<=t) two-tail	8.86E-09	
t Critical two-tail	2.306006	

Figure 4.33 Result of t-test exercise

Table 4.2 Explanations of some elements in t-test report

Mean	Measures of the average of a set of data (sometimes called 'arithmetic mean').
Variance	A measure of the spread of the values in a distribution. The larger the variance, the larger the distance of the individual cases from the group mean.

(*table continues overleaf*)

(Table 4.2 continued)

Observations	The number of data items.
Pearson Correlation	This is a correlation coefficient (parametric) test which measures the strength of a linear relationship between two random variables. Zero indicates variable independence; closer to 1 indicates greater linear dependence.
Hypothesized Mean Difference	We set this at the outset.
df	Degrees of freedom – the number of ways the data can be arranged, equal to 1 less than the number of pieces of data.
t Stat	The t Stat is a measure of how extreme a statistical estimate is. The hypothesised value (which we set to 0) is acceptable if the t Stat value is close to zero. If the t Stat value is positive, it suggests that the hypothesis value was not large enough (try again using a 1). If the t Stat is negative, it suggests that the hypothesis value was too large.
P(T<=t) one-tail	If t is greater than or equal to 0, the value of 'P(T <= t) one-tail' gives the probability that a value of the t-Statistic would be observed that is more positive than t. The opposite is true of a negative value here.

We have dealt here with a number of statistical tests, and hope that through trying these you build the confidence to try out others as your requirements present.

4.5 Graphs and charts

In this section we are going to look at charts as a visual aid to presenting data.

One of the great strengths of a spreadsheet is the ability to produce charts – for most of us, the visual information given by a graph or chart is easier to understand than a series of numbers. Rather than presenting numbers to support your discussion, a carefully prepared chart will instantly make the picture clear; more so than just words.

In healthcare we use charts a great deal: temperature, pulse, respiration and blood pressure charts; intake and output charts; and height and weight charts, to name just a few. We use these to help us see changes quickly. Spreadsheets can display changes in this way, but they can also display general results.

4.5.1 Creating charts in Excel

To demonstrate the process, we will start with a very simple column chart.

EXERCISE 4.14

1 Open a clean copy of *Demographic and health indicators.xls*. Highlight cells A34 to B38.

2 **Excel 2007**
Go to **Insert ➤ Charts** and click on the corner down-arrow to get the dialog box shown in Figure 4.34. Choose **Column** and the first (top left) of the icons, and press **OK.**

Figure 4.34
Chart options in
Excel 2007

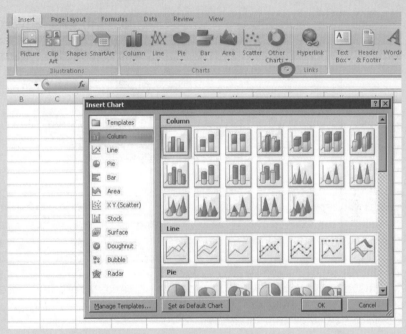

A chart will appear in the middle of your sheet and the Chart Tools toolbars will appear at the top of the Excel window. Look to the right of the **Design** toolbar, and you will see **Move Chart Location**. Left-click on this and choose to place your chart on a new sheet.

3 **Excel 2003**
❒ Go to **Insert ➤ Chart** and left-click to start the Chart Wizard (Fig 4.35).
❒ In Step 1, select **Column** as the Chart Type, and highlight the first (top left) of the Chart sub-types. Press **Next.**
❒ In Step 2, preview your chart; it should be set to 'Columns'. Press **Next.**
❒ In Step 3, you can do things like add a title and change various options, but we are going to come back to those later. Press **Next.**

❒ In Step 4, choose to place your chart on a new sheet. Press **Finish**.

A chart will appear in the middle of your new sheet, and the word 'Chart' will appear in the menu bar near the top of your Excel screen.

Figure 4.35
Chart Wizard in
Excel 2003

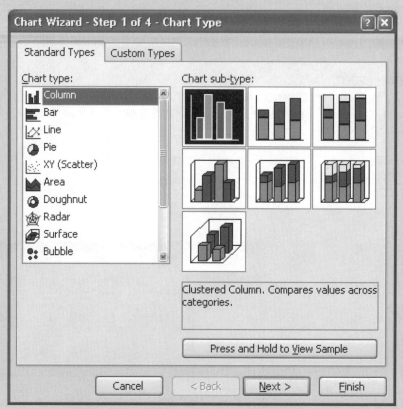

Now you have a chart upon which you can clearly see the gradual increase over the years. At the moment, however, this chart could be about anything, so we need to add labels to help with understanding.

4   The options for customising your chart are found in different places in Excel 2007 and Excel 2003 and work slightly differently, but they both do basically the same things.
    ❒ In Excel 2007, the options are found under **Chart Tools** in the **Layout** section.
    ❒ In Excel 2003, go to **Chart ➤ Chart Options** and a dialog box containing a number of tabs will open.

5   First we will add a title and axis labels to the chart.
    ❒ If you have the option, choose to resize the chart; otherwise this will be done automatically. Type in **Population Growth** as the Chart Title.
    ❒ For the horizontal axis (*x*-axis), type **Years 1976 to 1996**.
    ❒ For the vertical axis (*y*-axis), type **Population**.

6 To the right of your chart, you will see a box containing 'Series1' and a block the same colour as the columns. This is the 'legend' or 'key' for the chart. As we only have one series of data being represented we don't really need a legend, find the **Legend** options and remove it. Click on **OK**.

7 Now, left-click on one of the *y*-axis values to select that axis. Now right-click and choose **Format Axis**. Under **Number**, change the number of decimal places to zero. The final chart should appear as in Figure 4.36.

Figure 4.36
The final chart

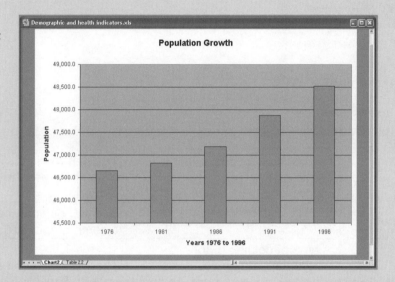

The last part of this exercise involves experimenting with different chart types – you might want to save your work so far first!

8 Try changing the column chart you created to a pie chart. In Excel 2007, look to the left of the **Design** section of the Chart Tools toolbar. In Excel 2003, go to **Chart ➤ Chart Type**. Find the section with pie chart options and choose one.

You will see that this type of chart really doesn't help with understanding these particular data. Try some of the others, and see what you think about their ability to clearly display the growth in population during this time period. You will probably find that a number of chart types help with displaying the numbers in a meaningful way, while there will be some charts that you cannot use as they require more than one series of numbers. Of which more later!

4.5.2   Chart types

As you can see, charts can be created really easily in Excel, but it helps to have some idea of what type of chart is best for what type of data. Table 4.3 summarises this information for the main types of chart. You can experiment to find out which of the other types are display your data clearly.

Table 4.3 Main chart types

Chart type	Use	Notes
Line	For continuous data, where points on the lines between the plotted points have a meaning.	You can read points off the graph between the ones you plotted.
Bar, column	For displaying data in categories.	Bar graphs are horizontal and column graphs are vertical.
Histogram	A type of column graph, where the data on the x-axis are grouped, and there are no gaps between the columns. Remember that this type of graph is used to show frequency distribution.	There is only one series of data. In Excel you can edit the 'Series1' options to take out the gaps produced in an ordinary column graph.
Pie	To show categories as part of a whole or to indicate percentages of a whole.	If you have a large number of categories, they can be hard to read, so showing the labels and percentages is a good option. Make sure that you are actually plotting parts out of 100 – it is easy to get this wrong and distort your data.
Scatter	To correlate one factor against another, i.e. to compare pairs of values.	Trend lines can be drawn through scatter plots to give a general correlation.

Charts should always have headings to explain what they are about, and labels on the axes or sections if these aren't self-explanatory. Otherwise, you can choose which options you want. Be aware that some of the effects available in Excel can distort your presentation of the data – this is particularly true of 3D effects, so use those cautiously.

4.5.3 Placing a chart into another application

You can also place a chart into any other Office application. Here's how.

Into a text document – Microsoft Word
In Excel, first select the entire chart. Then:

- in Excel 2007, go to **Home ➤ Copy** icon
- in Excel 2003, go to **Edit ➤ Copy**.

Now open Word – either open the document in which you want the chart to appear, or open a new document for test purposes. Then:

- in Word 2007, go to **Home ➤ Paste**
- in Word 2003, go to **Edit ➤ Paste**.

Your chart will now appear in the Word document.

Into a PowerPoint presentation
In Excel, first select the entire chart. Then:

- in Excel 2007, go to **Home ➤ Copy** icon
- in Excel 2003, go to **Edit ➤ Copy**.

Now open PowerPoint (either a presentation on which you are already working, or a new presentation for test purposes), and select a new slide (commonly a blank page) Then:

- in PowerPoint 2007, go to **Home ➤ Paste**
- in PowerPoint 2003, go to **Edit ➤ Paste**.

Your chart will appear on the slide.

Placing dynamic data
The above system works well when using published data that is not going to change, but sometimes the data may be dynamic – changes may be necessary which result in the need to update the image in the text or in the presentation. This can be done using the **Paste Special** command rather than the simple **Paste** command.

In Excel, first select the entire chart. Then:

- in Excel 2007, go to **Home ➤ Copy** icon
- in Excel 2003, go to **Edit ➤ Copy**.

Now open Word (either the document in which you want the chart to appear, or a new document for test purposes). Then:

- in Word 2007, go to **Home ➤ Paste Special**
- in Word 2003, go to **Edit ➤ Paste Special**.

In the dialog box, look to see that 'Microsoft Office Excel Chart Object' is highlighted, then select the check box next to **Paste link**. This will ensure that if we change the original data for the chart, our change will be reflected in this chart in this Word document.

Many Office applications are set to automatically update links when you open a file, but it is safest to manually update your links to be sure, before you finalise a presentation.

- To change options for updating links in Word, for example:
  - in Word 2007 go to **Office button ➤ Prepare** and scroll down to left-click on **Edit Links to Files**
  - in Word 2003, go to **Edit ➤ Links**.
- To do a manual update, change your chart in Excel and save. Go to the presentation containing the linked chart, select the chart, right-click and choose **Update Link**.

Your revised figures will appear in the chart.

Quick hint

When you paste, your chart may not be shown completely on your page or in your presentation. Click on the chart to get a box with small blocks (handles) on it. Grab one of the corner handles with your mouse and drag it into the middle to resize the chart. In some instances, where you are using a complex chart you might instead want to display it using a different orientation to your page, for example landscape instead of portrait.

EXERCISE 4.15 (SELF-STUDY)

1 Using a new spreadsheet, enter the following numbers in column B, rows 4 to 10, and save:

   34, 22, 23, 43, 33, 40, 18

   These represent the numbers of patients seen in your clinical unit over a seven-day period starting with Sunday. Prepare a suitable chart using these numbers to show variation of patient numbers over a week in your clinical unit. Do not close the spreadsheet file.

2 Place the chart you created in question 1 onto a Word page in a way that the original data can be changed; save this document. Do not close the Word file.

3 Return to the original (still open) Excel sheet. Change B5 to 34 and B10 to 38, and save the revised sheet. Now return to your (still open) Word document and update the link. Note what happens.

4.5.4 Charts using multiple data series

In section 4.5.1, we looked at building a chart using just one series of data; now we shall consider how to present multiple series of data.

Exercise 4.16

1 Open the spreadsheet *Population.xls* provided on the CD, and highlight G48 to M52. Note that for this example we have only used rows that contain data, and have thus left out 2006 as some data are missing. This would be explained in any commentary associated with the chart presentation.

2 **Excel 2007**
   ❏ In the same way as Exercise 4.13, go to the **Insert** ribbon and insert a plain Column chart. Move it to a new sheet.
   ❏ Under Chart Tools, go to the **Data** section and choose **Select Data**. Here is where we can change the default series labels to the years selected. Left-click on 'Series1' and press **Edit**; type 2001 in the white box labelled **Series name** and press **OK**. Now click on 'Series2', **Edit** and enter 2002; and so on until all are listed correctly.
   ❏ We also want to change the 1 to 7 on the *x*-axis. In the same **Select Data Source** box, look to the right to where it says 'Horizontal (Category) Axis Labels'. Left-click on **Edit**; the box will change to a smaller **Axis Labels** box. Move back to your spreadsheet (using the tabs at the bottom of the Excel window), and highlight cells G8 to M8; press **OK**. You will be bounced back into your chart, and will see that the labels have changed. (Note that you will have to manually edit out the unwanted superscripts on some of the country names – we will cover that later.) Press **OK**.
   ❏ Under the Chart Tools **Layout** tab, enter the chart title and axis labels as in Exercise 4.13. Name the chart 'Live Births in 7 European Countries'. The Category (X) axis box can be left blank, as (given the title) the labels are self-explanatory. Value (Y) axis should read 'Number of live births per 1000'.

3 **Excel 2003**
   ❏ In the same way as Exercise 4.13, start the Chart Wizard and choose a plain Column chart.
   ❏ In Step 2, first check that 'Rows' is selected in the **Data Range** tab (there should be five data series).
   ❏ Go to the **Series** tab. Here we can change the default series labels to the years selected. Highlight 'Series1' (it might be pre-selected) and type 2001 into the white box labelled **Name**. Next highlight 'Series2; and give it the name 2002; and so on until all are listed correctly. You will see the correct labels showing up in the legend on the little preview chart.

❐   We also want to change the 1 to 7 on the *x*-axis. Still in the Series tab, go
    down to the bottom to where it says **Category (X) axis labels**. Left-click
    on the small icon to the right of the white box, and then *on the spreadsheet*
    highlight cells G8 to M8. In the mini-dialog box that has popped up, left-click
    on the icon again. The '1 to 7' will change to the names of the counties.
    (Note that you will have to manually edit out the unwanted superscripts on
    some of the country names – we will cover that later.) Press **Next**.

❐   Under the **Titles** tab in Step 3, give the chart the name 'Live Births in 7
    European Countries'. The Category (X) axis box can be left blank, as (given
    the title) the labels are self-explanatory. Value (Y) axis should read 'Number
    of live births per 1000'. Press **Next**.

❐   In Step 4, select **As new sheet** and then press **Finish**.

Your chart is now ready for you to use it as you require. The chart should look
something like Figure 4.37.

To remove the unwanted numbers on some of the countries, you will have to go
back to the spreadsheet and edit out the numbers using the formula bar; the chart
will automatically update. Of course, by doing this you will be losing information
on the original spreadsheet, so it is always wise to first make a copy of your
spreadsheet file (giving it an appropriate name), and use your copy to create your
charts.

Figure 4.37
Multiple data
chart

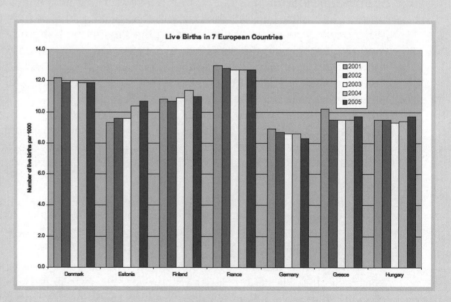

4   (Self-study) Once you have mastered the basics of using charts, try out different
    types to see if they present the data any more clearly than this easy column one
    we have used in this exercise.

5 Databases

Learning objectives

When this chapter is completed, you will be able to:

- understand the components of a database and how they can be used
- evaluate when a database is likely to be a tool suited to your information needs
- understand how to bring data into a database and to ask questions of that data
- develop reports from a database
- present data effectively from a database
- identify issues of data quality and develop strategies to improve the quality of health data
- understand common components of health data and the classifications used to represent health data.

This book is intended to help you build confidence in the use of health data. The most successful method for building understanding and confidence is to *do*.

To help you understand the material and to take in the concepts in this chapter, try to think as if the tasks have been given to you by your employer, and progress systematically through the tasks provided in each exercise. This approach is designed to give you experience in solving problems yourself, and to develop your confidence. There are times, just as in the real world, when you will find this challenging or difficult. Particularly when learning about databases, you will need to progress through several stages before the whole will be clear to you. If you feel that you need to complete a section more than once – do so. Remember that to learn we often need to move outside our comfort zone, and that you are developing new skills as well as new knowledge.

There are four exercises provided in this chapter. The data in the patient data files for these examples are of the same or similar structure to that collected in health systems all over the world, but are fictitious and do not represent any real patients. Exercises 5.1 and 5.3 are worked through in the book, and the screenshot examples follow these. Exercises 5.2 and 5.4 are associated practice exercises. These follow the same general path as the other exercises, but are intended to be self-directed. Details of each exercise are given overleaf.

Exercise 5.1

- For this exercise, the file *Cardiovascular cases for the year.csv* is provided on the CD. This file represents patients treated for cardiovascular problems in your area.
- You have been asked to identify the difference in prevalence of disease and age group of the people represented in this file according to whether they are smokers or not. The text will explain all of the steps required to achieve this goal, and you should carry out those steps in your own copy of the database as you work through.
- This task will also require the files *Diagnosis Codes.csv* and *Procedure Codes.xls*.
- Completed databases of this exercise are provided for reference, called *Cardiovascular cases 1.mdb* (to Step 29) and *Cardiovascular cases 2.mdb* (for steps 30 onwards).

Exercise 5.2 *(SELF-STUDY)*

- This is similar to Exercise 5.1 in the steps to be followed, but is based upon a different file of data. In this case the file is called *Cancer cases for the year.csv*.
- You are asked to find the difference between rates of cancer for people admitted from suburbs in the north and north-east, to those admitted from the south and south-east, comparing the ages and suburbs of the patients.
- You should complete each activity for Exercise 5.2 after each step outlined using Exercise 5.1. These steps indicate the tasks you should complete for this self-directed task.
- A completed database of this exercise is provided so that you can use it to assist you if needed; it is called *Cancer cases.mdb*.
- This task will also require the files *Diagnosis Codes.csv* and *Provider Codes.csv*.

Exercise 5.3

- This exercise requires you to build a database of your own to collect data about patients waiting for treatment.
- Details to be added to the database are provided, and a complete solution is provided in the database called *Waiting List.mdb*.

Exercise 5.4 *(SELF-STUDY)*

- This self-directed exercise aims to give you practice in developing your own database to collect and analyse information.
- In this case you are to develop a data collection system for people attending a community centre so that these patients may be sent follow-up letters to remind them of the need for a pap smear. A complete solution is provided in the database called *Recalls.mdb* and the files *Recall letter template.doc* and *Recall letter result.doc*.

The complete set of developed databases for all four exercises is provided on the CD for you to review.

5.1   The basics

To understand databases and to complete the tasks used to build your confidence and skills, in addition to this book and the associated CD/website you will need to understand how computers do some of the things they do. Not at the detailed programming level, but at a level that gives you the capacity to control the information you receive and have to manage.

5.1.1   What is a database and why would I use one?

A database is like a box that holds cards upon which you have stored information. You may sort the cards in many different ways, and you can pull out the cards that meet certain criteria – for example those for people who are female or those with a specific disease. A database works well like this – *provided* that the data are suitably organised and recorded in a manner that can be processed by a computer.

At this point it is vital to realise just how 'stupid' the computer is. If you asked a person to look in the box and pull out all the cards for women, that person would be able to understand your intention; they would pull out each card that indicated a person as 'female', or 'sex = F', or 'woman', or even symbols used to represent the concept of gender. A computer, however, requires a more consistent representation of data. In order for the computer to pull out all the cards for women, the indication of gender would have to be done the same way on every card – for example *all* 'female' or *all* 'sex = F', but not a mixture of both.

A database is a file that includes data and the relationships between those data; databases may also include programs for extraction (queries/reporting) or presentation (reporting) of data and the support of data collection (screens/forms). A file that simply contains data is not usually referred to as a database. Such files include .csv files (comma-separated variables or values) and spreadsheets.

Databases are designed to handle:

- complex data – data that have a number of foci; for example, data about people and their disease conditions
- large amounts of data – as they make the management and analysis of that data simpler
- data of which questions should or could be asked, but where those questions are not yet well defined
- data that needs to be processed – aggregated, counted or retrieved by different field values. For example, data where you might wish to find out information today according to a particular disease, and tomorrow by people's financial status. A card box, unfortunately, is limited to a single-sort sequence – a database is not.

5.1.2   Getting started

To use data, you must first know where to find the necessary information, and be able to evaluate the content of the information available. The first steps in the exercises below involve copying the relevant .csv file to your local machine or storage device. You must think clearly about where you will files the database file you will create. The original .csv files contain a large amount of data, and once this is stored as a database the size of the database file will increase as you use it. As a rule of thumb, you need at least three times the size of the file available as free space in the area in which you plan to file it.

EXERCISE 5.1

First, find the data. The files are stored on the CD.

1   Copy *Cardiovascular cases for the year.csv* to an appropriate folder/directory on your own hard disk. Then copy the two files *Diagnosis Codes.csv* and *Procedure Codes.xls* to the same location.

2   What size is each of these three files?

You will also need to think about how and where to backup your work on the database. Section 2.4.1 runs through the most common options along with their advantages and disadvantages. See also the important information about saving in section 5.2.3.

EXERCISE 5.2 (SELF-STUDY)

1   Copy the exercise file *Cancer cases for the year.csv* and the background files *Diagnosis Codes.csv* and *Provider codes.csv* to your hard disk.

2   What size is the file *Cancer cases for the year.csv*?

5.2   Introduction to Access

When you get started with any new area of knowledge, there is always new terminology with which you must become familiar. While all database products have similar functions, this book uses Microsoft Access as a learning tool. This is simply because this is the most commonly available tool of its kind. It does not imply that this is the best or recommended data collection tool; in fact, most healthcare organisations have significantly more powerful systems available. However, once you are familiar with the capacity and processes for manipulating data in one database system, you will find that the same general principles apply to all others. All can collect and store data; all can query and select specific data according to your instructions; and all can report upon the data.

Access is a Relational Database Management System (RDBMS). RDBMSs provide:

- storage for the data
- tools that help with the management of that data
- more specific tools that assist you in extracting data and developing visually appropriate or Web-based data entry screens.

This type of software product has been developed so that you do not have to be a programmer to use the system. The system provides an interface that 'hides' the fact that software is actually being written as you use the tools. There is sufficient flexibility that Access (and similar software) can be used to develop simple systems. It may also be employed by more advanced users in association with more sophisticated programming languages to produce a more complex result, but we will not cover that functionality here.

5.2.1   Starting Access

Starting (also called launching or opening) Access can be achieved in a number of ways. The method you choose is likely to be influenced by the way your computer has been set up. In all cases, Access can be started by going via the Windows Start menu:

- **Start ➤ Programs ➤ Microsoft Office ➤ Microsoft Access** (2007 or 2003).

When you open Access, you see the 'empty' Access screen shown in Figure 5.1 (overleaf).

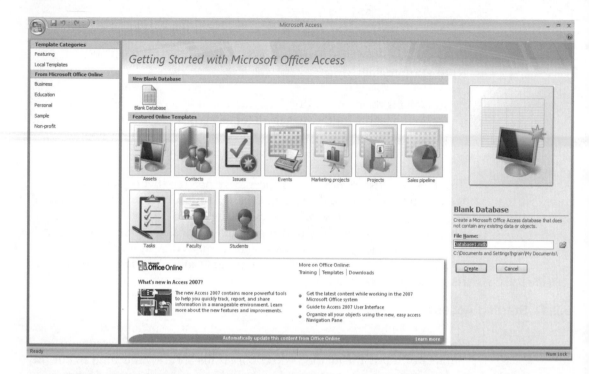

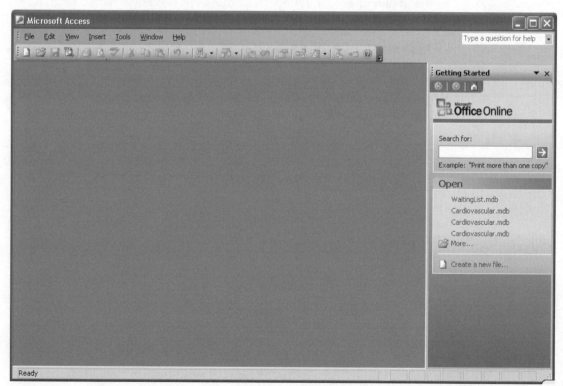

Figure 5.1 Initial screen in (top) Access 2007; (bottom) Access 2003

5.2.2   Creating a new database

The starting file *Cardiovascular cases for the year.csv* is not a database file but a .csv file – this stands for comma-separated variables (or values). Each different piece of data in that file is separated by a comma, and each new record/entry in the file has a return (enter) symbol at the end. If you opened the file without any structure, it would look like Figure 5.2.

1285,1,M,I841,,,,,,,,,,,,,,,,,,,,,3209000,9250300,,,,,,,,,,,,Y,10,6

824,2,M,I269,G4732,,,,,,,,,,,,,,,,,9203800,9555009,,,,,,,,,,,N,10,6

878,1,M,I352,I10,,,,,,,,,,,,,,,,,,,3821800,5992100,,,,,,,,,,,Y,10,8

881,2,F,I208,I2511,Z951,Z955,E780,I10,,,,,,,,,,,,,,,,3821800,5990000,,,,,,,,,,,N,10,6

Figure 5.2 Comma-Separated Variables/Values file structure

If you double-click on this file, it will open up in a spreadsheet. But we want to import these data into a database. This requires specific instructions to the system. First, you need to create a database into which you can put the information.

Look at your opening screen.

- In Access 2007, on the bottom right is a section called **Blank Database** (Fig 5.3). This is where you can create a new, empty database. Give your database a name, and left-click on **Create**.
- In Access 2003, to the right there is a **Getting Started** panel. Left-click on **Create a new file**.

This will bring up the **New File** panel on the right of the screen (Fig 5.4).

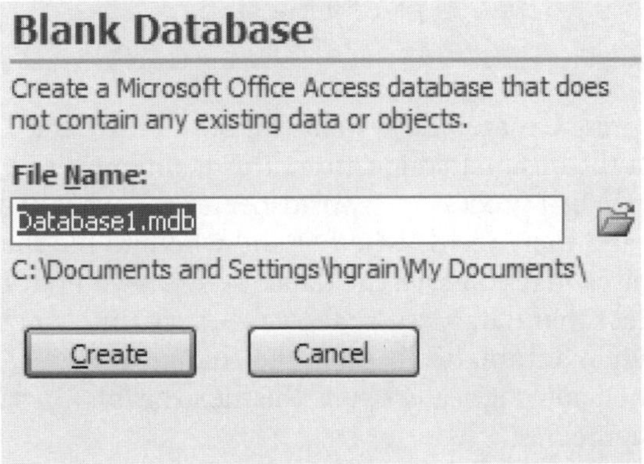

Figure 5.3 Blank Database screen in Access 2007

Blank Database

Create a Microsoft Office Access database that does not contain any existing data or objects.

File Name:

Database1.mdb

C:\Documents and Settings\hgrain\My Documents\

Create   Cancel

Figure 5.4
New File panel

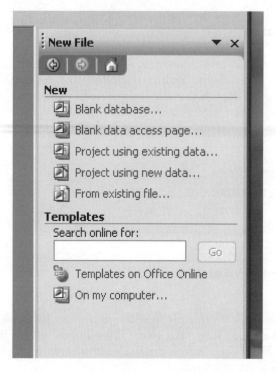

The **New File** panel gives you the option to create a new file without any existing structure, or to use a standard structure from a pre-existing template. We want a blank database.

EXERCISE 5.1 CONTINUED

Open Access if it is not open already.

3 Create a new file with the name *Cardiovascular.mdb* and chose to place it in the same folder or directory where you placed the starting files.

When you press **Create**, the system will both create the new database and file it in the designated location. This is different to most other types of software (Word processors, spreadsheets etc), where you create new documents and then decide whether and where to file them or save them. Access requires that you save the database *before* you put data into it. This is due to the fact that databases 'self-save' – every time you add new data to the files, the system automatically saves the change.

Access then automatically opens the file. The 'blank' database screen is shown in Figure 5.5.

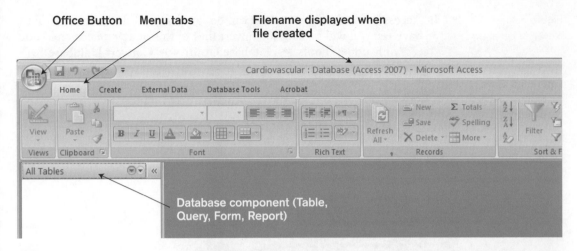

Office Button   Menu tabs   Filename displayed when file created

Figure 5.5
Blank database content screen in (top) Access 2007; (bottom) Access 2003

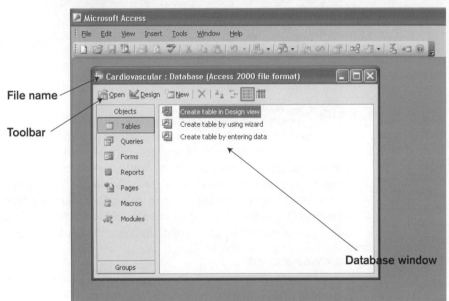

Database component (Table, Query, Form, Report)

File name

Toolbar

Database window

5.2.3 Saving your database files

It is important to realise that an Access database holds not just files of data (called tables), but also files of program instructions for queries, forms, reports, etc. The database will automatically save new records created in tables, and you will be prompted to save changes to program instructions files (where the design instructions for tables, queries, forms and reports are held) when you make them.

- In Access 2007, use **Office Button ➤ Save ➤ Save As** to save the *current object* in the database (such as a table or a report), or to convert the database to another copy in the same format or a previous version (Fig 5.6).

- In Access 2003, the *current object* can be saved using **File ➤ Save** or **File ➤ Save As**; you will be able to convert files to this or a *previous* version of Access only under **Tools ➤ Database Utilities ➤ Convert Database**.

Figure 5.6 Save As Options in Access 2007

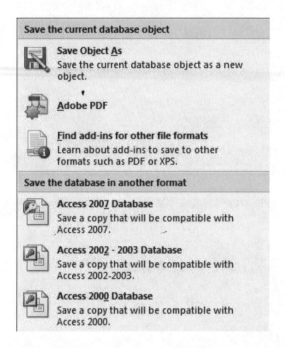

It is important to recognise that, unlike most types of file, you *cannot* use the **Save As** option with Access *for the full database*. You must close the database, and then copy the file and change its name if you want to make a copy or backup. To make a backup of your database, copy the file to an alternative device and give it an appropriate name; you should do this regularly.

5.2.4 Finding your way around

Access 2007

Figure 5.7 shows the menu tabs as you see them when you first open Access 2007, i.e. with the Home ribbon showing. The icons are not active until a database table has been created. When first opened there are no tables or data in the system, so the icons on the Home ribbon are largely inactive and appear greyed out.

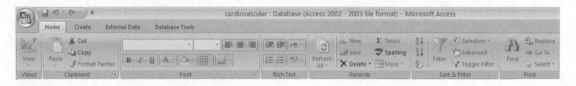

Figure 5.7 Home ribbon showing greyed-out icons

There are four general menus under the tabs in Figure 5.7: Home, Create, External Data, and Database Tools. It is worth spending some time looking at each of these to get familiar with what they offer, even if you don't know what the functions do. They will be introduced as we use them in the worked examples below.

Database window

This window, found on the right of the Access 2007 screen (Fig 5.8), provides details of the content of the database, and allows you to launch specific activities such as design modifications to Tables, Queries, Forms or Reports, or to create new objects (Tables, Forms or Reports).

Figure 5.8
Database screen components, Access 2007

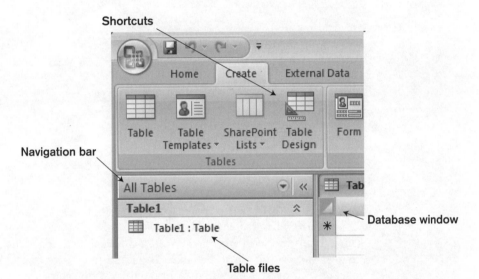

The menu options and actions you will be offered will differ depending on what type of object you are working with, and the way in which you are viewing it. For example, if you are looking at the Design View of your data, you will be offered menu options to do with managing and manipulating that data; if you are in Datasheet View you will be shown the actual data (or report or form), and the menu options will change accordingly. There is more about the different database views in section 5.3.2.

Navigation Pane

The Navigation Pane, to the left, lists the objects available in your database. You can use the down-arrow to the right of the navigation bar to select other object types to view what else is filed within the database. These object types include:

- Tables – which hold your data
- Queries – which hold instructions for data extraction and calculation and the data resulting from those instructions
- Forms – the design of screens for data capture and display
- Reports – the design and resulting data for presentation of data in reports.

If you left-click the double arrows on the right of the Navigation Pane the whole object display section will close so that you can see more of the data view. Figure 5.9 shows the Navigation Pane closed. Note that until there is data in tables in your database, any actions in the menu ribbon that require data will appear greyed out (inactive).

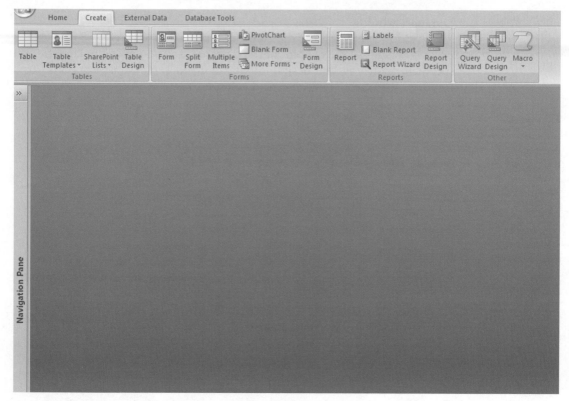

Figure 5.9 Database screen with Navigation Pane closed

Access 2003

When you create a new database or open one in Access 2003, a new Database window opens up in your Access screen (Fig 5.10).

Figure 5.10
Database view in
Access 2003

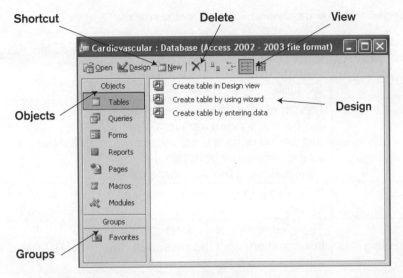

The main (white) window provides details of the content of the database, and allows you to create new objects. The object types are listed in the panel on the left:

- Tables – which hold your data
- Queries – which hold instructions for data extraction and calculation and the data resulting from those instructions
- Forms – the design of screens for data capture and display
- Reports – the design and resulting data for presentation of data in reports.

Any new objects you create will appear in the main window. Left-clicking on each heading in the left-hand panel will bring up a list of created objects in the main window.

5.3   Importing and using tables

Tables are the files in the database that hold the actual data. You will need to bring the three files provided to you into the database: to do this, you will need to *import* each of the files from the CD.

Before you do this, however, you should understand the purpose of and the data included in each of the files. Table 5.1 indicates the data elements included in the file *Cardiovascular cases for the year.csv*.

Table 5.1 Data elements in *Cardiovascular cases for the year.csv*

Data element	Description	Values or codes used
Record ID	A unique identifier of each entry in the table	Number
LOS	Length of stay (the number of days the person was an inpatient during this period of care – calculated as the difference between the admission and the discharge dates)	Number
Sex	Indicates if the person is male or female	M = Male F = Female
Principal Diag	The diagnosis which, after investigation, was the reason for the admission to hospital	ICD10-AM diagnosis code
Other Diag01 to Other Diag25	Other diagnosis, complications, causes of injury, place of occurrence of injury, activity when injured, health status (including smoking status) and injuries	ICD10-AM diagnosis code
Proc01 to Proc15	Procedures and treatments undertaken during the hospitalisation	ICD10-AM procedure code
sameday	Indicates where the episode of care was for a single day (admission and discharge dates are the same)	Y = this case is sameday N = this case is not sameday
Suburb	Indicates the area in which the individual lived at the time of admission to the hospital	10 = Northern 11 = North Eastern 12 = Eastern 13 = South Eastern 14 = Southern 15 = South Western 16 = Western 18 = North Western 19 = Central
Age Group	The age group into which the individual falls on the day of admission	0 = 0–9 1 = 10–19 2 = 20–29 3 = 30–39 4 = 40–49 5 = 50–59 6 = 60–69 7 = 70–79 8 = 80–89 9 = 90 or over

As shown in Table 5.1, the data indicates the values in all data elements except those represented by detailed diagnosis or procedure codes. These codes are based on the World Health Organization's International Classification of Diseases (ICD).

The two additional data files provided indicate the code and the description of that code. Both tables have the same structure – see Table 5.2.

Table 5.2 Data elements in *Diagnosis Codes.csv* and *Procedure Codes.xls*

code_ID	The actual ICD code (as recorded in the Diagnosis or Procedure fields in the *Cardiovascular cases for the year* data table), e.g. A020
ascii_desc	The description that explains what the code standards for, e.g. Salmonella enteritis

It is important to note that the codes used in these tables are from the Australian version of ICD10, called ICD10AM. The code system and the rules used to allocate codes are updated regularly in most countries – and the tables provided here should only be used for the purposes of the exercises. If you need to use these codes in your local environment, you should obtain a copy of the codes and descriptions relevant at the time of the data collection in your local system.

5.3.1   Importing data

To bring the data from each file into the database so that you can work on them you must import them one at a time.

EXERCISE 5.1 CONTINUED

4   First import *Cardiovascular cases for the year.csv*.
   ❐ In Access 2007, go to the **External Data** ribbon (Fig 5.11). Choose **Import ► Text File**. This will bring up the dialog box shown in Figure 5.12.

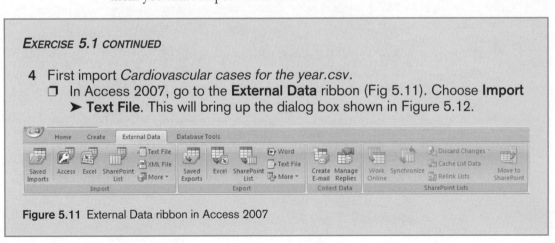

Figure 5.11 External Data ribbon in Access 2007

Figure 5.12
Import text
dialog box for
Access 2007

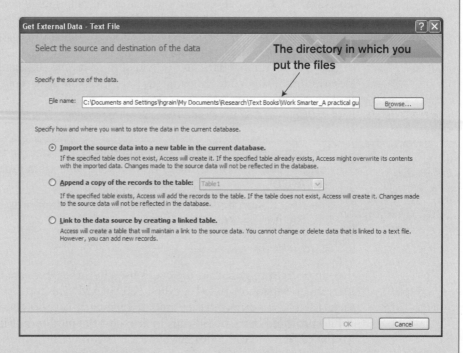

Select the directory in which you have stored the files. If you cannot remember the whole string of folders and filenames, use the **Browse** option to find the .csv file.

There are also options on whether you want to put the data into a new table, add it to an existing table, or leave the data in the original file and use Access to get the data out of that original source each time you want to view/add/modify the data.

☐ Choose to create a new table that holds the content from the file (i.e. 'Import the source data into a new table in the current database.').
   Ensure the file *Cardiovascular cases for the year.csv* is selected and click on **OK**.
☐ In Access 2003, ensure that you have **Tables** selected in the database dialog box, then go to **File ➤ Get External Data ➤ Import**. This will bring up the dialog box shown in Figure 5.13.

Figure 5.13
Import text dialog
box for Access
2003

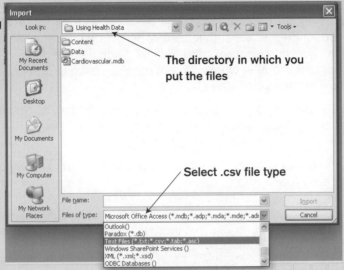

☐ Change **Files of type:** to Text Files, and find and select *Cardiovascular cases for the year.csv.* Press **Import**.

This will start the Import Text Wizard, which will look at the contents of the file to be imported and assist you to set up the file with appropriate fields (Fig 5.14).

Figure 5.14
Import Text
Wizard,
showing file
structure

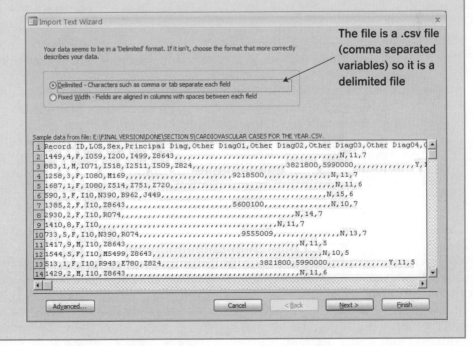

When importing a file there are two options.
- ❏ The file can have a special character that is used to indicate where a new data element begins (as in this case, where a comma is used to indicate the start of a new data element or to 'delimit' each field of data).
- ❏ The other alternative is where the data are in columns and have a consistent width or size throughout the file.

The computer system identifies which file type this is likely to be and will default to the most appropriate option (in this case the delimited option). The bottom half of the Wizard box shows a sample of the data.

5 Having ensured that delimited is selected, press **Next** to get the next screen in the Import Text Wizard (Fig 5.15).

This shows the effect of the delimiter (in the bottom part of the screen) and allows you to select another character (e.g. a tab) as the delimiter if you are not getting the correct result. In this instance, the use of a comma clearly puts data into defined fields with a heading at the top.

Ensure that 'First Row Contains Field Names' is selected (to properly identify the heading), and press **Next**. In Access 2003, you will be given the option to store the data in a new table or an existing table; choose 'In a New Table' and press **Next**.

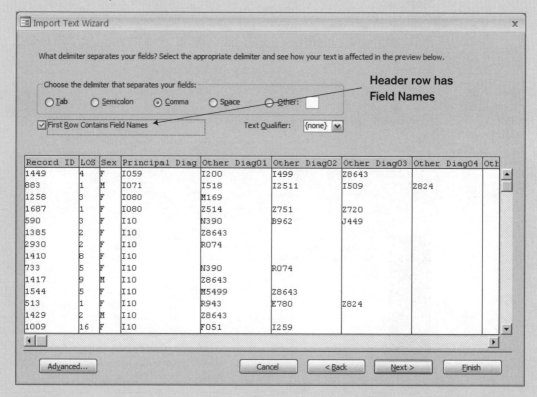

Figure 5.15 Import Text Wizard, showing Field Names

You will now get the screen shown in Figure 5.16. Having determined each field name, the system displays how the resulting table will look, and allows you to change the technical structure of the data. This is an issue that is discussed later (section 5.10).

Figure 5.16
Field options in the Import Text Wizard

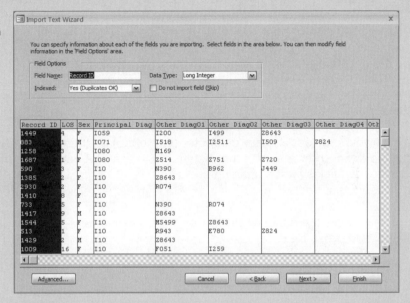

6   This time, there is no need for any modifications to the computer's suggestions. Press **Next**. You will get the screen shown in Figure 5.17.

Figure 5.17
Selection of the primary key

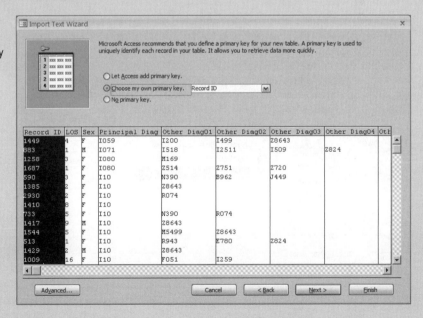

In a database the computer uses a 'primary key' to uniquely identify each individual entry in a table. In the case of *Cardiovascular cases for the year.csv*, the **Record ID** should be selected as the primary key – the screen will have defaulted to plain 'ID'.

7   As shown in Figure 5.17, select 'Choose my own primary key', and choose **Record ID**. Then press **Next**.

8   The last decision to be made when importing a file is what name you will give the new table being created. The system will automatically use the same name as the original file used to import the data. You may change this if you wish (Fig 5.18). Press **Finish**.

Figure 5.18
Naming the new table

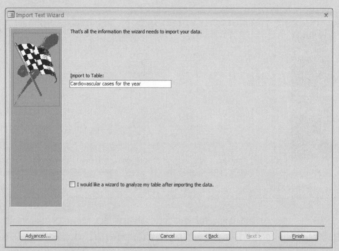

When you press **Finish**, the system will give you a message confirming that the data have been imported, then return you to the general database window – which is now showing the new file (Fig 5.19).

Figure 5.19
Database window showing imported file (Access 2003)

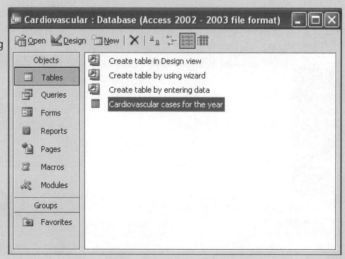

9 In a similar way, import the two additional files, *Diagnosis Codes.csv* and *Procedure Codes.xls*, noting the following differences:

- ❒ For the .xls file, you will need to choose the file type Microsoft Excel.
- ❒ For both files, the **code_id** field should be chosen as the primary key.

When you have finished, the database window will show all three files.

Quick hint

When you import files from other sources, you should always check to ensure that *all* records have come into the new database. You should ask the provider of the files the number of records that are in each file, and compare this with the number of records in the tables established in the database. The correct record numbers for the tables provided in this book are:

Cardiovascular cases for the year	3,423
Cancer cases for the year	2,775
Diagnosis Codes	15,914
Procedure Codes	5,926

10 Check the numbers of records in each of your imported files against the numbers shown in the Quick hint box.

5.3.2 Views of data

To look more closely at (for example) the *Cardiovascular cases for the year* table, you can open the table. There are two ways to look at a table: you can look at the *content* of the table or the *structure* of the table.

To look at the content, simply double-click on the Table name or select the table and press the **Open** icon. You will get the window shown in Figure 5.20 (overleaf), known as the Datasheet View.

The scroll bars at the right and bottom of the table show that there are more fields and rows than are seen in the window. The Datasheet View shows the components of the table, and also indicates the number of records in the table. There are icons at the bottom left for moving through the records to modify and view data.

**Rows (records)
with data**   **Table name**   **Field**

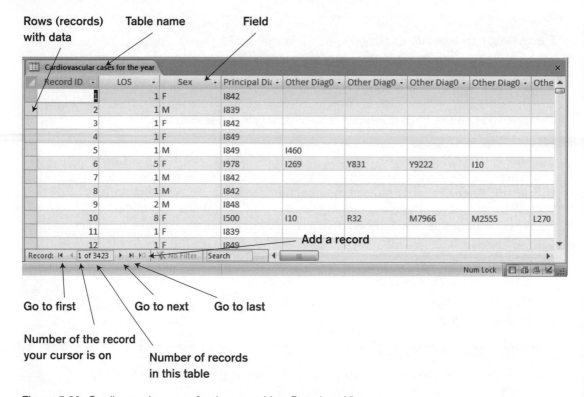

Record ID	LOS	Sex	Principal Dia	Other Diag0	Other Diag0	Other Diag0	Other Diag0	Othe
1	1	F	I842					
2	1	M	I839					
3	1	F	I842					
4	1	F	I849					
5	1	M	I849	I460				
6	5	F	I978	I269	Y831	Y9222	I10	
7	1	M	I842					
8	1	M	I842					
9	2	M	I848					
10	8	F	I500	I10	R32	M7966	M2555	L270
11	1	F	I839					
12	1	F	I849					

Add a record

Record: ⊮ ◂ 1 of 3423 ▸ ▸⊮ ▸⊱ ☒ No Filter | Search

Num Lock

Go to first   **Go to next**   **Go to last**

**Number of the record
your cursor is on**   **Number of records
in this table**

Figure 5.20 *Cardiovascular cases for the year* table – Datasheet View

When you have a table open in the Datasheet View, the toolbar changes,
showing different icons. In particular, the icon at the far left becomes a View
icon (Fig 5.21) which you can use to switch between different views.

Figure 5.21
View icon and
view options

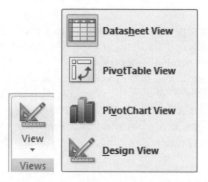

To see the range of fields available in the database and the size and type of
each field (the field table structure), you must change to the Design View of
the data.

EXERCISE 5.1 CONTINUED

11   In your main database window, double-click to open the Datasheet View of the
table *Cardiovascular cases for the year*. Left-click on the **View** icon and choose
Design View. Your view will change to the Design View (Fig 5.22), and the View
icon will change to the Datasheet View icon.

The Design View shows every field in the table along with the structure and
rules that apply to that field.

Name of each field

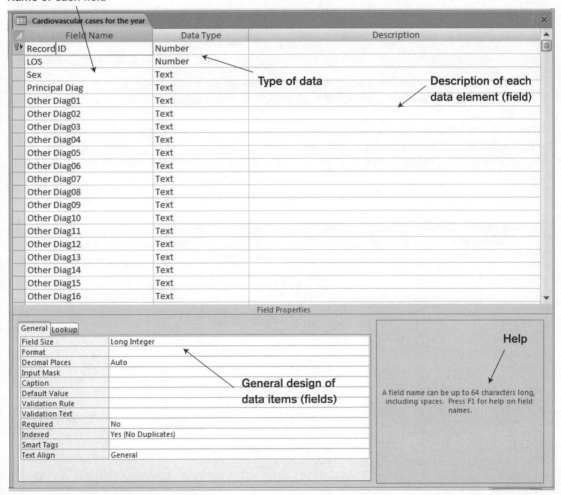

Figure 5.22 Design View for tables

For example, in Figure 5.23, the first field is the Record ID; this field is a
number, and it holds the unique identifier for the record in the table – it is
the primary key, indicated by the small key icon in the far left column.

The Data Type column indicates the type of data held; what type of data is specified puts in place some rules about the content of the field. For example, Record ID is a number. If you tried to add a new record with a Record ID of ABC123 the computer would not let you – as ABC123 is not a number. Data types are discussed in more detail later, as we work through the exercise.

The Description column is a free-text field, used to indicate what the field is used for. Although the description has no control over the structure of the item itself, it is of great value in helping you – and others – remember what the data in the field represents. The data in this table were imported automatically from a file which did not contain descriptions. (The commas in the descriptions would have altered the structure of the table – wrongly – when the data were imported.)

EXERCISE 5.1 CONTINUED

12 In Design View for the table *Cardiovascular cases for the year*, left-click in the description area and type in each description, as shown in Figure 5.23.

Note: if you have descriptions in a different computer file (word-processor, spreadsheet or database), you can copy and paste them from there into the appropriate description area. A copy of Table 5.1 is provided on the CD for you to use.

Field Name	Data Type	Description
Record ID	Number	A unique identifier of each entry in the table
LOS	Number	Length of Stay (the numb er of days the person was an inpatient during the period - calculat
Sex	Text	Indicates if the person is Male or Female
Principal Diag	Text	The diagnosis which, after investigation was the reason for the admission to hospital
Other Diag01	Text	Other diagnosis, complications, causes of injury, place of occurrence of injury, activity wher
Other Diag02	Text	Other diagnosis, complications, causes of injury, place of occurrence of injury, activity wher
Other Diag03	Text	Other diagnosis, complications, causes of injury, place of occurrence of injury, activity wher
Other Diag04	Text	Other diagnosis, complications, causes of injury, place of occurrence of injury, activity wher
Other Diag05	Text	Other diagnosis, complications, causes of injury, place of occurrence of injury, activity wher
Other Diag06	Text	Other diagnosis, complications, causes of injury, place of occurrence of injury, activity wher
Other Diag07	Text	Other diagnosis, complications, causes of injury, place of occurrence of injury, activity wher
Other Diag08	Text	Other diagnosis, complications, causes of injury, place of occurrence of injury, activity wher
Other Diag09	Text	Other diagnosis, complications, causes of injury, place of occurrence of injury, activity wher

Cardiovascular cases for the year

Field Properties

General | Lookup

Field Size	Long Integer
Format	
Decimal Places	Auto
Input Mask	
Caption	
Default Value	
Validation Rule	
Validation Text	
Required	No
Indexed	Yes (No Duplicates)
Smart Tags	
Text Align	General

Indicates more specifically the data type

Not a required field

A field name can be up to 64 characters long, including spaces. Press F1 for help on field names.

Figure 5.23 Design View of table, with Descriptions fields completed

You can see *how* the Data Type control the structure and content of the data by looking at the information provided in the **General** and **Lookup** tabs. For example, Figure 5.23 shows the **General** tab information for Record ID (indicated by black arrow in the left-hand column). This shows that Record ID is a Long Integer and is not a Required Field, i.e. it doesn't have to be entered for every record. You don't need to know more about this now; later on in the book we will go into table design in more detail.

Note that when you click on a field name, the details in the **General** tab change to reflect the structure of the data element you have selected. In the **General** tab, if you then left-click on 'Long Integer' the screen on the right (containing blue type) will display Help details to explain 'Long Integer' (Fig 5.24). If you then move down to the next row you will get Help information on 'Format'; and so on down the screen.

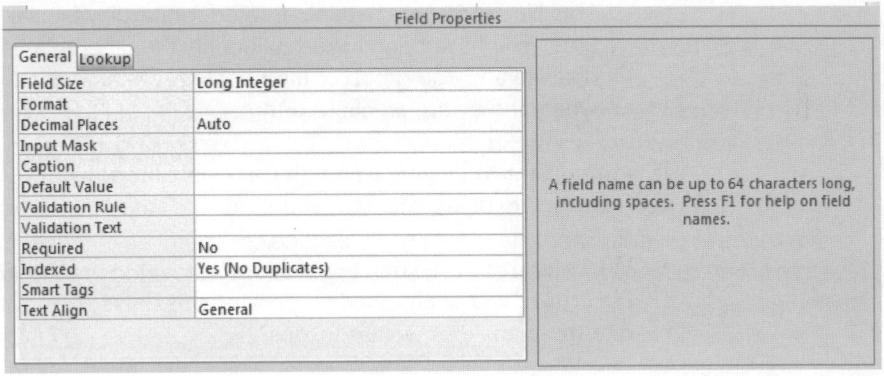

Figure 5.24
General field structure and associated Help

Field Properties		
General | Lookup		
Field Size	Long Integer	
Format		
Decimal Places	Auto	
Input Mask		
Caption		
Default Value		A field name can be up to 64 characters long, including spaces. Press F1 for help on field names.
Validation Rule		
Validation Text		
Required	No	
Indexed	Yes (No Duplicates)	
Smart Tags		
Text Align	General	

If you left-click on space alongside 'Default Value' in the **General** tab, the Help information provided is:

A value that is automatically entered in this field for new records

A common default value in healthcare is the use of 'today's date' in the Admission Date field, or the date of visit or service provision. This is a useful concept that can both save time in entering data, and also improve the quality of the data when a field has a consistent value that can be defined in rules such as 'use today's date'.

EXERCISE *5.2* (SELF-STUDY) CONTINUED

3 Import the files *Cancer cases for the year.csv*, *Diagnosis Codes.csv* and *Provider Codes.csv*, and enter the descriptions relevant for each field.

4 Check the number of records in each file. These should be:

Cancer cases for the year	2,775
Diagnosis Codes	15,914
Provider Codes	5,926

5.4   How queries work

Queries are questions asked of the database. The questions can be stored, and asked again and again as data changes. You can copy a question and make changes to it. The ability to ask questions of a database is one of its main strengths.

5.4.1   The question

In order to ask a question of a database, however, you must understand *exactly* what the question is. We need to look again at what Exercise 5.1 is asking us to do with the file *Cardiovascular cases for the year*:

> This file represents patients treated for cardiovascular problems in your area. You have been asked to identify the difference in prevalence of disease and age group of the people represented in this file according to whether they are smokers or not.

It is important to be able to break this question down into components that you can specify using the data and structure that you have. For example:

- What figures have you been asked for?   *Prevalence*
- How have you been asked to present this data?   *By disease and age group*
- Are there any special conditions?   *(1) Smokers/non smokers*
                                            (2) In your area

For each of these components, you need to identify *how* you will calculate or identify each element.

Prevalence

What is meant by *prevalence*? In this instance you have figures that represent episodes of care in hospital. The records in the table, although constructed from individuals' visits to hospital, represent those *individual visits*, not the individual person. There is no way to tell from the data collection if a single person came in more than once during the period: there is no unique person identifier in the data collection, just a unique record ID. Therefore, this data set could never be used to calculate a person- or population-based representation of disease in a community. It *can* represent the services provided for different diseases and age groups.

If asked to provide prevalence information, you would need to confirm with the requestor that the information you can provide will meet their need.

Disease

Does this mean *anyone* who had a cardiovascular condition? Look at the table *Cardiovascular cases for the year* – all diagnosis codes that start with an 'I' are circulatory system codes. The only cases contained in the original data file are for people admitted to hospital for circulatory system problems; all such problems have a code in the Principal Diagnosis field starts that with an 'I'.

The meaning of each code can be found by looking it up in the appropriate code table. For example, if you want to know what the value 'I10' in the Principal Diagnosis field means:

- open the Diagnosis Codes table and select the **code_id** column by left-click anywhere in that column. Then:
    - in Access 2007, go to **Home ➤ Find**
    - in Access 2003, go to **Edit ➤ Find**. The Find and Replace dialog box will open (Fig 5.25).

Figure 5.25
Searching for 'I10'

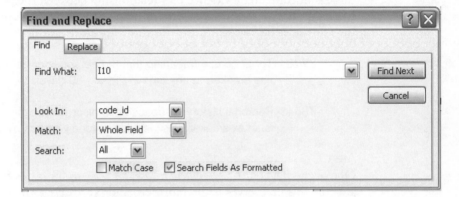

- In the **Find What** section you enter the value you are looking for (search criteria).
- In the **Look In** section you indicate the field in which the computer is to search.
- **Match** indicates whether you want the computer to: match your search criteria *exactly* (whole field); just find your criteria somewhere in the field (part of field); or find results only where your criteria are at the start of the field.
- Press **Find Next**, and the table view will go to the first case of your criteria in the code_id field (Fig 5.26).

Figure 5.26
Result of search on 'I10'

code_id	ascii_desc
I082	Disorders of both aortic and tricuspid valves
I083	Combined disorders of mitral
I088	Other multiple valve diseases
I089	Multiple valve disease
I090	Rheumatic myocarditis
I091	Rheumatic diseases of endocardium
I092	Chronic rheumatic pericarditis
I098	Other specified rheumatic heart diseases
I099	Rheumatic heart disease
I10	Essential (primary) hypertension
I110	Hypertensive heart disease with (congestive) heart failure
I119	Hypertensive heart disease without (congestive) heart failure

To complete any task that has to retrieve disease data from a database, you must understand exactly which diseases you want to include, and whether it is the disease that caused the admission (a condition in the Principal Diagnosis field) or any disease in the other 24 disease fields.

Smoker?

How will you identify if the person represented by the record in the database is a smoker or not? Try doing a search on the word 'tobacco' in the ascii_desc section of the *Diagnosis Codes* table. There are two basic types of 'disease' code here. The first F170–F179 covers smoking as a mental disorder (related to dependence or harmful use) – this code is generally only used when there is documented evidence of a relationship between the condition and smoking. The most common form of indicating smoking status is through the two codes below:

> Z720   Tobacco use (meaning that the person is currently smoking or has smoked at any time in the last 30 days).

> Z8643   Personal history of tobacco use disorder (meaning that the person is an ex-smoker; this includes anyone who has ever smoked).

Area

One of the fields in *Cardiovascular cases for the year* indicates Suburb. The area the hospital serves is the Northern and North Eastern area. Therefore you must only include records that have the values 10 or 11 in the Suburb field. These are the codes representing the Northern and North Eastern suburbs (look back to Table 5.1, page 168, where the codes for the suburbs are provided).

Now back to the question. To answer the initial request, you will need to determine exactly how you will define that request, to frame a question. Often the requestor's requirements seem clear until you start to specify *exactly* what is wanted, look at the data available, and try to work out how you will meet the request.

You should identify what information you can provide, and clearly define it. Here is the definition of what we will provide in response to the question we have been asked in Exercise 5.1:

> The number of episodes for people with cardiovascular disease from the northern or north-eastern suburb by 10-year age groups (because the only age groups available in the database are 10-year groups).

The components are defined as:

- *Cardiovascular disease* – any record that has an entry in the Principal Diagnosis field that begins with an 'I'.
- *Smoker/Non-smoker* – any record with either Z720 or Z8643 in any of the Other Diag fields will be counted as a smoker; records without such codes will be counted as non-smokers.
- *Area* – any record where the Suburb code is 10 (northern) or 11 (north-eastern); the suburbs will not be reported on individually.

When you have decided on your question, you need to confirm it with the requester.

EXERCISE 5.2 *(SELF-STUDY) CONTINUED*

You have been asked to find the difference between rates of cancer for people admitted from suburbs in the north and north-east, to those admitted from the south and south-east, comparing the ages and suburbs of the patients.

5 What is your question? Consider the way you will define 'cancer', and the data you need to include to work out where a person lives and the rate of cancer.

5.4.2 Creating a new query

Databases use queries to extract data from tables (or from existing queries). The queries are used to define which fields are to be included in the extracted data, and to restrict and sort the data obtained. They are the computer's way of asking questions.

The steps required to represent a question should be done one by one. Build a query that meets your first criteria – check it; then add another element of your criteria – check that; then add another element. In this way you know that if the answer provided by the query no longer fits your question, the error is in your last change. To develop a query for our Exercise 5.1 question defined above, the steps will be:

Step 1 Include only the fields required
Only include the Principal Diag, Age Group (which will be seen in the report), and the Other Diag and Suburb fields, as these will be needed in Step 2.

Step 2 Include only the records needed (restrict the records to those relevant to the question)
For cardiovascular disease, include any record that has an entry in the Principal Diag field that begins with an 'I'.

For area, include any record where the Suburb code is 10 (northern) or 11 (north-eastern).

Step 3 Identify which are smokers and which non-smokers
Include any record with either Z720 or Z8643 in any of the Other Diag fields.

To do this, you create a new field that indicates whether the entry represents a smoker. (If it doesn't, this field will be blank.) This will take several query stages. The first will be to find all the records that have either of the codes required in any of the Other Diag fields. Once you have these cases, you need to create a new field to indicate that each person found is counted as a smoker. There are many ways to do this – the method used here will be to create a new copy of the data that holds just the fields necessary to answer the question.

EXERCISE 5.1 CONTINUED

13 To create a new query which you can design to obtain the information you need:
   ❑ In Access 2007, go to the **Create** ribbon (Fig 5.27), then **Other ➤ Query Design.**
   ❑ In Access 2003, select the **Query** object in the left-hand panel of the main database window, and double-click on 'Create query in Design View'.

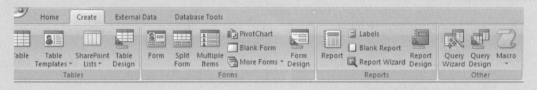

Figure 5.27 Create ribbon in Access 2007

After you have initiated the new query design, you will be asked to select the table(s) on which the query is to be based (Fig 5.28). This dialog box gives you the option to add any tables or (queries that already exist) to the selection of data for this new query.

Choose to add the file which you have determined is the one required to answer our question, *Cardiovascular cases for the year,* by selecting it and either pressing **Add** or double-clicking.

Figure 5.28
Show Table
dialog box

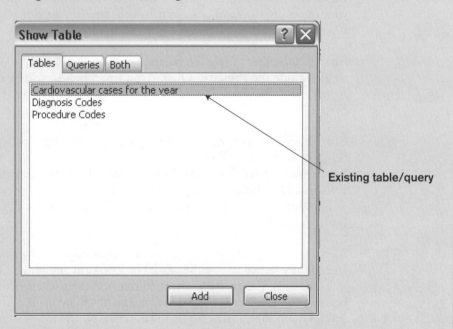

Existing table/query

As you click on each table or query you need, they will be added to the Select Query window (Fig 5.29). It is called 'Query1: Select Query' because it is actually a query used to select data items from one or more established tables and/or queries.

After closing the Show Table dialog box, you can change the size of the Select Query box (both main window and the different halves) or the small Table box inside it in the normal way (by clicking and dragging to the size required).

Figure 5.29
Select Query window showing Query design grid

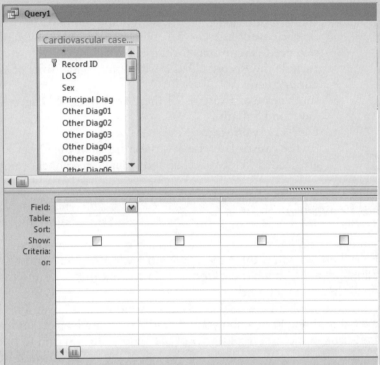

Figure 5.30
Datasheet View icon

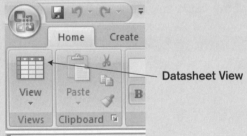

Having selected the table (the first step), if you now choose the Datasheet View icon in the toolbar (Fig 5.30) you will get an error message:

Query must have at least one destination field.

This message reflects the fact that you haven't yet told the new query which fields to include.

5.4.3 Adding fields to the query

You need to consider which fields you will need in your query, and put each of them into the Field section of the Query Design grid.

The fields you should include in a query are those you need to:

* *See in the final data*
  (in the case of Exercise 5.1, these are Principal Diag and Age Group. We also need descriptions for those two fields).
  Include the Record ID as it is the unique identifier of each entry.
* *Use as criteria*
  (in the case of Exercise 5.1 these are Principal Diag, which we already have, and Suburb).
* *Use for calculations*
  (in the case of Exercise 5.1, these are all of the Other Diag fields – which are needed to identify if an individual is a smoker or not).

EXERCISE 5.1 CONTINUED

14 Add the required fields to the Query Design grid. You can do this in three ways:
  ☐ Find the field you want in the small table window (scroll down as necessary). Highlight it and double-click on it. This will put that field into the next empty field position in the grid.
  ☐ Find and highlight the field in the table window as above, then left-click and drag it to the field position you want in the Query Design grid.
  ☐ Left-click in the first (Field) row of the Query Design grid to bring up show a drop-down arrow, and use this to select the field you want from the list of available fields. Move on to the next Field space and repeat.

Figure 5.31 shows some of the fields selected.

Figure 5.31
Selection of data items for query

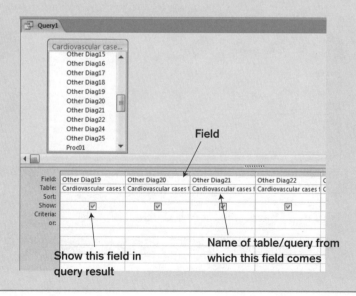

15 As you do each step of a query (or any other programming activity), you should always check that you have achieved what you intended. To do this, go to the Datasheet View to see the data you have extracted.

You will notice that *everything* is showing – not just the data items we wish to show. We also still have the same number of records as we did when we began, as we haven't restricted the suburbs or diseases yet.

❐ Go back to Design View, and remove the check mark from the **Show** boxes on those fields that you would not need to see in the final Query file (Fig 5.32), then return to Datasheet View to check (Fig 5.33).

Note that the data items appear in the same sequence as in the columns of the Query Design grid.

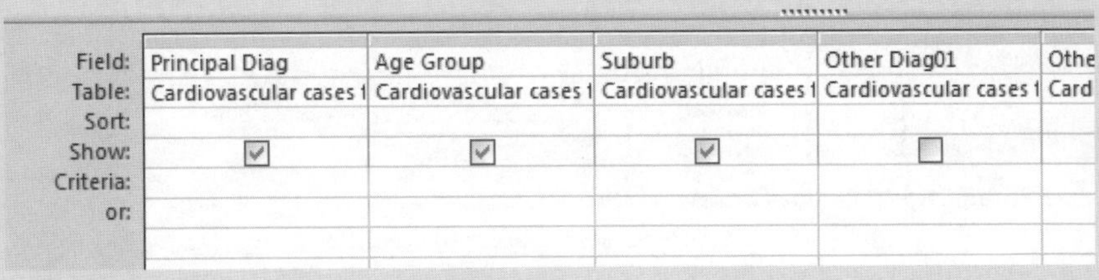

Figure 5.32
Removing check marks on fields not needed to be shown in the final result

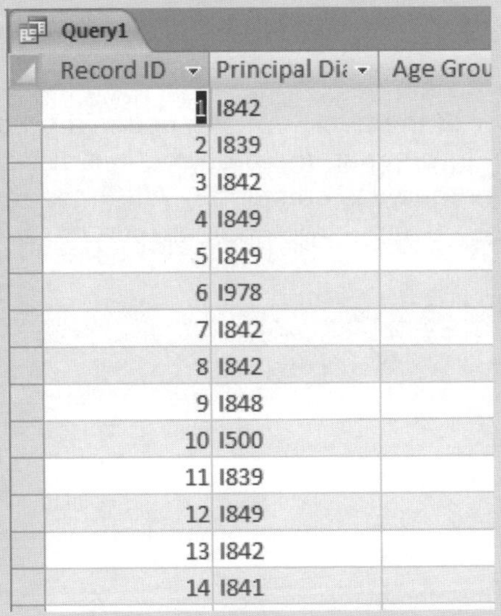

Field:	Principal Diag	Age Group	Suburb	Other Diag01	Othe
Table:	Cardiovascular cases 1	Cardiovascular cases 1	Cardiovascular cases 1	Cardiovascular cases 1	Card
Sort:					
Show:	☑	☑	☑	☐	
Criteria:					
or:					

Figure 5.33
Datasheet View of fields selected

Query1

Record ID ▾	Principal Dia ▾	Age Grou
1	I842	
2	I839	
3	I842	
4	I849	
5	I849	
6	I978	
7	I842	
8	I842	
9	I848	
10	I500	
11	I839	
12	I849	
13	I842	
14	I841	

16 Regular saving after checking of each change, using appropriate names for your objects, is strongly recommended. If you are happy that your query includes the data you want, you should save it. Give it the name *Smokers/Non Smokers*. (If you want, you may now close the query and return to it later.)

17 Although your query table (as shown in Fig 5.33) contains the Record ID, Principal Diag and Age Group fields, the result is not showing the descriptions for the diagnosis codes. This requires the inclusion in the query of the descriptions from the *Diagnosis Codes* table.

To add this table to your query, you need to re-open the Show Table window (Fig 5.28). To do this, return to the Design View of the query, then:

❏ in Access 2007, go to **Query Tools** ribbon ➤ **View** ➤ **Design**, then right-click and choose **Show Table**

❏ in Access 2003, go to **Query** ➤ **Show Table** or click on the **Show Table** icon in the toolbar.

Add the *Diagnosis Codes* table to the query, and close the Show Table window. The Query Design window will now look like Figure 5.34.

Figure 5.34
Query Design window containing two tables

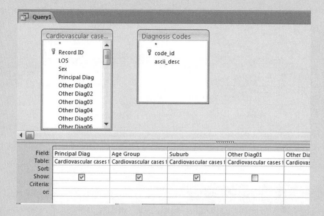

If you now go to the Datasheet View of the query you will notice a problem. It will take a *very* long time for the system to bring up the record count at the bottom of the screen (this is how you know that the query is complete). When the record count does finally appear, it is 54,473,622 – a very large number (see Fig 5.35).

Figure 5.35
Result of unrelated multiple table query

Record ID	Principal Dia	Age Group	Suburb	Other
1449	I059	7	11	Z8643
883	I071	7	13	I509
1258	I080	7	11	
1687	I080	6	11	Z720
590	I10	6	15	J449
1385	I10	7	10	
2930	I10	7	14	
1410	I10	7	11	
733	I10	7	13	
1417	I10	5	11	
1544	I10	5	10	
513	I10	5	11	Z824
1429	I10	6	11	

Record: I◀ ◀ 1 of 54473622 ▶ ▶I ▶ 🏷 No Filter | Search

The original *Cardiovascular cases for the year* table had 3,243 records. A query on that table should *never* have more entries than that. What has happened is that after you add the second file to the query, the computer tries to apply the query to every record in both files. The record count in your query is thus the total number of records for the cardiovascular table *multiplied by* the total number of records in the diagnosis table!

To solve this problem, you must establish a *relationship* between the tables. This allows the computer to 'know' that the Principal Diag field contains codes that have the same values as the entries in the *Disease Code* table's code_id field.

5.4.4 Relationships

Quick hint

If you're not sure which are the fields that hold the same information, open each table in the Datasheet View and see what the data look like. You can also check the Design View of the tables – the items should be the same size and type.

Relationships indicate where tables share a common piece of information that can be used to link from one table to the other. In our example, the *Cardiovascular codes for the year* and *Diagnosis Codes* tables both have a field which contains the ICD10 code, although the fields have different Field Names – Principal Diag in one table, and code_id in the other table.

Figure 5.36 shows the relationship established between the Principal Diag field (for which you want to display the code description) and the code_id field (which holds the same values Principal Diag and offers the link to the ascii_desc field that gives the code description).

Figure 5.36
Relationship between like fields

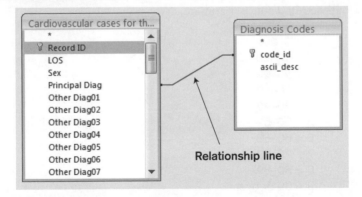

EXERCISE 5.1 CONTINUED

18   To create a relationship you need to build a link between the Principal Diag
field in the *Cardiovascular cases for the year* table and the code_id field in the
Diagnosis Codes table. Note that relationships built in queries exist only in that
query, and are not applied elsewhere.

❒ In the Design View of your query, left-click on one of the fields to be linked,
drag that field over the top of the second field, and let go. This will put a line
between the two data items, as shown in Figure 5.36, linking them.

❒ You can now add the ascii_desc field to the query by left-clicking and
dragging it from the *Diagnosis Codes* table to the column in the query table
grid next to the Principle Diag column. (The other columns will shift to the
right to make room.)

To make sure it has worked correctly, look at the Datasheet View (Figure 5.37).
The descriptions will be visible – and you will be back to 3,423 records!

Record ID	Principal Dia	ascii_desc	Age Group	Sub
1449	I059	Mitral valve disease	7	
883	I071	Tricuspid insufficiency	7	
1258	I080	Disorders of both mitral and aortic valves	7	
1687	I080	Disorders of both mitral and aortic valves	6	
476	I10	Essential (primary) hypertension	6	
1426	I10	Essential (primary) hypertension	6	

Figure 5.37 Descriptions displayed after tables have been linked

The next step is to look at the Age Group fields – this is a code, not the
actual value of the age group. To correct this, you need to create another
table that can provide the descriptions for the Age Group codes in a similar
way to the code descriptions. The Age Group codes and descriptions were
outlined in Table 5.1 and are:

0 = 0–9
1 = 10–19
2 = 20–29
3 = 30–39
4 = 40–49
5 = 50–59
6 = 60–69
7 = 70–79
8 = 80–89
9 = 90 or over

Before you try to create a new table to hold these values, you need to decide
what fields will need to be in that table. Like the *Diagnosis Codes* table, this
new table needs two fields: the first to hold the code (we'll call it Age Code),
and the second to hold the description of that code (Age Description).

Quick hint

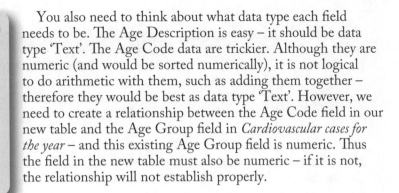

Only use data type 'Number' when you want the computer to be able to do arithmetic with the results, or where a relationship is required with a field that is numeric.

You also need to think about what data type each field needs to be. The Age Description is easy – it should be data type 'Text'. The Age Code data are trickier. Although they are numeric (and would be sorted numerically), it is not logical to do arithmetic with them, such as adding them together – therefore they would be best as data type 'Text'. However, we need to create a relationship between the Age Code field in our new table and the Age Group field in *Cardiovascular cases for the year* – and this existing Age Group field is numeric. Thus the field in the new table must also be numeric – if it is not, the relationship will not establish properly.

EXERCISE 5.1 CONTINUED

19 Create a new table to provide the Age Group descriptions. Left-click in the main database window, then:
- ❑ in Access 2007, go to **Create ➤ Table**
- ❑ in Access 2003, ensure that **Tables** is selected, then double-click on 'Create table in Design view' (or use the **New Object** icon and choose **Table** then **Design View**).

You will get a blank Table form (Fig 5.38). Enter the field name for each data element and the appropriate data. Set the Age Code to be the primary key, by left-clicking anywhere in the Age Code line and then right-clicking and selecting **Primary Key**.

The completed new table can be seen in Figure 5.39.

Figure 5.38
Empty table
in Design View

Figure 5.39
New entries
in table

Age Group Codes : Table		
Field Name	Data Type	Description
🔑▶ Age Code	Number	Code used for age groups
Age Description	Text	Description relevant to each age group code

20 Save this table under the name *Age Group Codes*, and close the window. The saved table will be visible in the main database window (Figure 5.40).

Figure 5.40
Age Group Codes table in database window

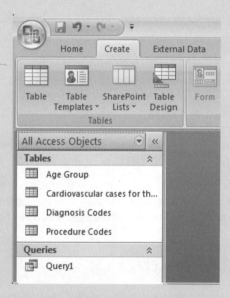

21 Now you need to add the codes and descriptions to the *Age Group Codes* table.
- ❐ Open the table by double-clicking on its name in the list on the main database window. This will open the table in the Datasheet view, ready to have data entered (Fig 5.41).
- ❐ Each field is displayed as the same size. To make it easier to use, click and drag out the right side of the Age Description column, then enter the data (Figure 5.42). Use the tab and return (enter) keys to move through the table as you type. When you are finished, close the table and save when prompted.

Figure 5.41
Empty table ready for data entry

Age Group Codes : Table	
Age Code	Age Description
▶	

Figure 5.42
Age Group
descriptions
entered

Age Group Codes : Table	
Age Code	Age Description
0	0 - 9
1	10 - 19
2	20 - 29
3	30 - 39
4	40 - 49
5	50 - 59
6	60 - 69
7	70 - 79
8	80 - 89
9	90 and over
*	

22 Remember the reason why this table was created? It is here to provide Age
Group descriptions for the query. To access these descriptions, there are three
things to do:
❐ insert the table into the query
❐ create a relationship between the Age Group field in the *Cardiovascular
   cases for the year* table and the Age Code field in the new table
❐ add the Age Description field to the fields in the query.

If you can do this without looking at the instructions that follow, do so – but if
you're not sure, follow the instructions below. When you have finished, save the
query.

To insert the table into the query:
❐ In the main database window, open the **Smokers/Non Smokers** query in
   Design View.
❐ Bring up **Show Table**, and add the *Age Group Codes* table to the query.
❐ Scroll down to find the **Age Group** field in the *Cardiovascular cases for the
   year* table, select it, and click and drag it to the **Age Code** field in the *Age
   Group* table. (Remember that you must only create relationships where the
   contents of the fields are the same.)

You should end up with links as shown in Figure 5.43.

Figure 5.43
Relationships
from the
*Cardiovascular
cases for the
year* table

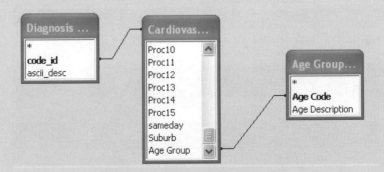

To check that your query still works properly, go to the Datasheet View. If it displays without any error messages the relationship has been appropriately created.

Return to the Design View. Add the Age Description field to the table by left-clicking and dragging it from the *Age Group* table to the column in the Query Table grid next to the Age Group column. (The other columns will shift to the right to make room.) You will see the screen shown in Figure 5.44.

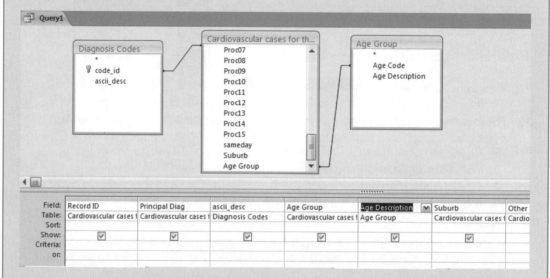

Figure 5.44 Age Description added to the query

Go to the Datasheet View to check that this has worked properly (Fig 5.45). Save the query.

Record ID	Principal Di	ascii_desc	Age Group	Age Descrip	Su
1449	I059	Mitral valve disease	7	70-79	
883	I071	Tricuspid insufficiency	7	70-79	
1258	I080	Disorders of both mitral and aortic valves	7	70-79	
1687	I080	Disorders of both mitral and aortic valves	6	60-69	
476	I10	Essential (primary) hypertension	6	60-69	
1426	I10	Essential (primary) hypertension	6	60-69	
1566	I10	Essential (primary) hypertension	8	80-89	
1125	I10	Essential (primary) hypertension	6	60-69	
1545	I10	Essential (primary) hypertension	7	70-79	
157	I10	Essential (primary) hypertension	6	60-69	
1746	I10	Essential (primary) hypertension	5	50-59	
1016	I10	Essential (primary) hypertension	7	70-79	

Figure 5.45 Age Description in Datasheet View of the query

We have now completed Step 1 in the process of answering our question.

5.4.5 Restricting the data to meet your criteria

Step 2 in the process of answering our question is to include only the records needed (restricting the records to those relevant to the question). For Exercise 5.1, that means that we only want cases that:

- are cardiovascular disease – any record that has an entry in the Principal Diag field that begins with an 'I'
- have a Suburb code of 10 (northern) or 11 (north-eastern).

This process is sometimes called *filtering*.

---

23 First, we restrict the data to cases with cardiovascular conditions in the Principal Diag field. To do this you must enter a criterion – in the **Criteria** row of the Principal Diag field – which specifies that the Principal Diag code must start with an 'I'.

  ❏ Open the *Smokers/Non Smokers* query and go to Design View. In the 'Principal Diag' column, left-click in the **Criteria** box and type I*. The '*', often called the wildcard, means to match anything; in this case, anything after the 'I'.

When you type I* and press enter, the computer will automatically format the 'syntax' (computer grammar) of the statement so that Access understands what you mean. It will become **Like "I*"** (Fig 5.46).

Figure 5.46
Wildcard
criteria

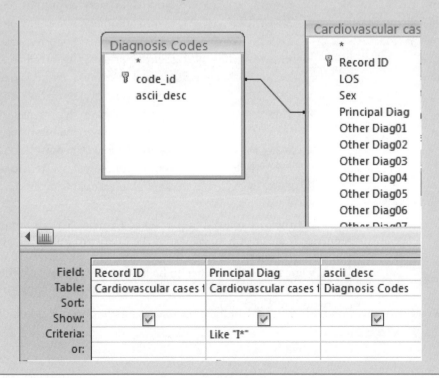

24 Now check that the entries in the Datasheet View match the criteria expected.
In Datasheet View, left-click anywhere in the Principal Diag column, then sort the data:

☐ in Access 2007, go to **Home** and look in the **Sort & Filter** section for the **Sort** buttons
☐ in Access 2003, there are two **Sort** buttons in the toolbar.

One button sorts ascending order:

The other sorts descending order:

First sort from top to bottom, and then from bottom to top. The first and the last entries should all begin with I (Figure 5.47).
If you are happy that you have the data you need, save the query.

Figure 5.47
Sorting the query
to check the
criteria

Record ID	Principal Diag	ascii_desc
1449	I059	Mitral valve disease
883	I071	Tricuspid insufficiency
1258	I080	Disorders of both mitral and aortic valves
1687	I080	Disorders of both mitral and aortic valves
62	I10	Essential (primary) hypertension
1545	I10	Essential (primary) hypertension
2484	I10	Essential (primary) hypertension
2746	I10	Essential (primary) hypertension
1575	I10	Essential (primary) hypertension
1585	I10	Essential (primary) hypertension
726	I10	Essential (primary) hypertension
1385	I10	Essential (primary) hypertension
1428	I10	Essential (primary) hypertension
1425	I10	Essential (primary) hypertension
592	I10	Essential (primary) hypertension
2758	I10	Essential (primary) hypertension

Note that the sort you did in part 24 of Exercise 5.1 is a temporary sort sequence that is not held as part of the query program. This means that if you close the query and open it again, the sort sequence will not be retained. If you want the sort sequence to be kept as part of the way the query always functions, you can include the Sort instruction in the appropriate row of the query design (Fig 5.48).

Figure 5.48
Adding a sort
sequence to the
query design

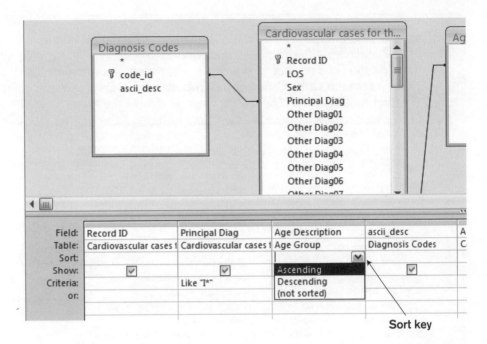

Sort key

Table 5.3 gives a list of example criteria entries that you may find useful.

Table 5.3 Example criteria entries

Field	Example	Meaning
Sex	M	Restrict records retrieved to those that = M
Sex	"M" or "F"	Retrieves any entry that is either M or F in the sex field
LOS	➤5	Retrieve only records that have a length of stay greater than 5
LOS	➤=10	Retrieve only records that have a length of stay equal to or greater than 10
Principal Diag	Like "I!"	Restrict records to those that start with I and have only one other character. (This is different to * which retrieves everything that starts with I irrespective of how many other characters there are)
Principal Diag	➤="I10" and <= "I259"	Retrieves all values between the two entries (including the entry values)
Proc01	Is null	Retrieves all records where the field Proc01 is empty
Proc02	Is not null	Retrieves all records where the field Proc01 is not empty

---

EXERCISE 5.1 CONTINUED

25 The second requirement is to include only those records with Suburb codes of 10 or 11. In the **Criteria** box of the Suburb field in Design View, enter **10 or 11** (Fig 5.49). Check it in Datasheet View, and save the query.

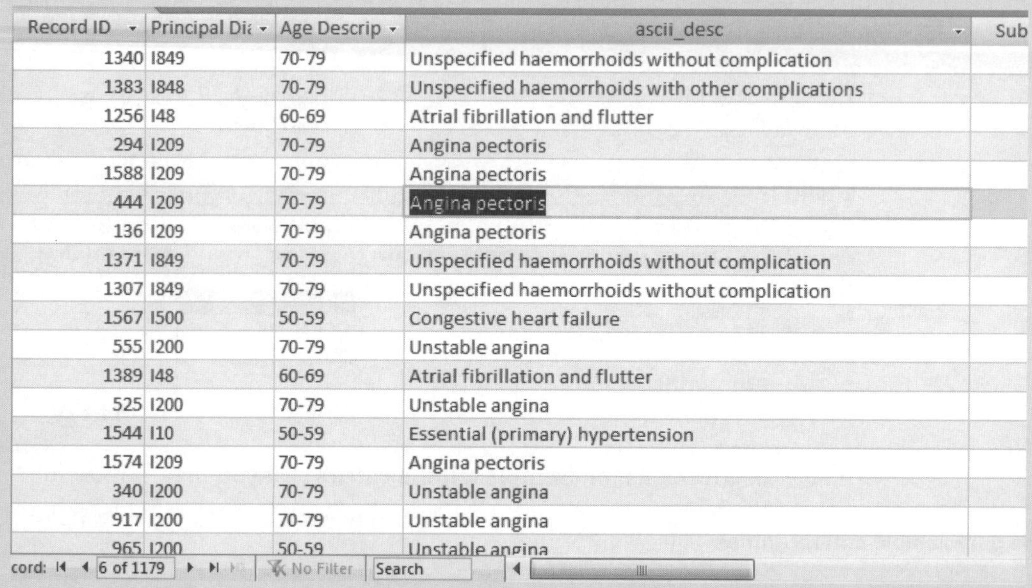

Record ID ▾	Principal Dia ▾	Age Descrip ▾	ascii_desc ▾	Sub
1340	I849	70-79	Unspecified haemorrhoids without complication	
1383	I848	70-79	Unspecified haemorrhoids with other complications	
1256	I48	60-69	Atrial fibrillation and flutter	
294	I209	70-79	Angina pectoris	
1588	I209	70-79	Angina pectoris	
444	I209	70-79	Angina pectoris	
136	I209	70-79	Angina pectoris	
1371	I849	70-79	Unspecified haemorrhoids without complication	
1307	I849	70-79	Unspecified haemorrhoids without complication	
1567	I500	50-59	Congestive heart failure	
555	I200	70-79	Unstable angina	
1389	I48	60-69	Atrial fibrillation and flutter	
525	I200	70-79	Unstable angina	
1544	I10	50-59	Essential (primary) hypertension	
1574	I209	70-79	Angina pectoris	
340	I200	70-79	Unstable angina	
917	I200	70-79	Unstable angina	
965	I200	50-59	Unstable angina	

cord: ◄ ◄ 6 of 1179 ► ►I ►   ⚑ No Filter   Search   ◄ ▒▒▒▒▒▒▒ ▒

Figure 5.49 Suburb restriction in Datasheet View

EXERCISE 5.2 (SELF-STUDY) CONTINUED

You have been asked to:

> Find the difference between rates of cancer for people admitted from suburbs in the north and north-east, to those admitted from the south and south-east, comparing the ages and suburbs of the patients.

In the steps below, remember to check each step by viewing the data after each step. That way you can more easily identify if you are doing the right thing and identify where you may have made an error.

6 Select the relevant tables to add to your query, and select the fields from those queries that you need to either represent or restrict the data needed.

7 Ensure that relationships have been properly set between the tables. Use the Datasheet View to see if the data looks correct (though you haven't yet restricted it to only cancer cases). Save after this step – if you view the data earlier the result will be an enormous file as the lack of relationships will build a match between all entries in all tables on all occasions.

8 Include the restriction to cancer cases only. Use the Datasheet View to see if the data looks correct: correct descriptions of the diseases and a smaller number of cases than you had in the previous version.

5.4.6 Multiple processes for a single result

The data needed to answer the question are now in the query, but the smokers are not yet clearly identified. To do this, we need to store the results in a way that we can make a report.

To complete this part of the information requirements, you need to derive a field from the information available – this involves multiple steps. Before you can make the necessary modifications to the query, you need to work out *how* to find the smokers. You only have to find one group (the smokers), as those who are not in that group are (of course) the non-smokers. The steps we need to take are:

- Find the smokers (add smoking to the query).
- Record that they are smokers – by creating a new field – and file the field appropriately.
- Create a new table that holds smoking status.
- Fill the table with smokers, then add the non-smokers to get a table from which we can produce the required report.

Finding the smokers

To find the records of smokers, you must look for any Other Diag fields which contain either the code Z720 (current smoker) or the code Z8643 (ex-smoker).

EXERCISE 5.1 CONTINUED

26 To find the records of smokers, either current or ex, open the query *Smokers/ Non Smokers* in Design View and type **Z720 or Z8643** into the **Criteria** box of Other Diag01 (Fig 5.50). Access will put in the quote marks for you.

Field:	Record ID	Principal Diag	Age Descriptic	ascii_desc	Suburb	Other Diag01	O
Table:	Cardiovasc	Cardiovascular cases 1	Age Group	Diagnosis Codes	Cardiovascular cases 1	Cardiovascular cases 1	Ca
Sort:							
Show:	✓	✓	✓	✓	✓	✓	
Criteria:		Like "I*"			10 Or 11	"Z720" Or "Z8643"	
or:							

Figure 5.50 Selection of smoking cases in Other Diag01

This results in a Datasheet View that is limited to only 72 records (Fig 5.51).

Query1

Principle Di	Age Group	Expr1002	Age Description	Suburb	Other Diag0
I848	6	60 - 69	60 - 69	11	Z720
I7021	7	70 - 79	70 - 79	10	Z720
I848	7	70 - 79	70 - 79	10	Z720
I7023	5	50 - 59	50 - 59	10	Z720
I7023	6	60 - 69	60 - 69	10	Z720
I7020	7	70 - 79	70 - 79	11	Z8643
I840	6	60 - 69	60 - 69	11	Z720
I839	8	80 - 89	80 - 89	11	Z8643
I849	5	50 - 59	50 - 59	11	Z720
I839	7	70 - 79	70 - 79	10	Z720
I200	5	50 - 59	50 - 59	11	Z8643

Record: 7 of 72 No Filter Search

Figure 5.51 Result of 'Smoker' restriction in Other Diag01

Step 26 of Exercise 5.1 partly meets the requirements. To find *every* person who is or was a smoker, you need to add the same criterion to all of the Other Diag02 to Other Diag25 fields. However, it is not as simple as adding the criterion to the rest of the Other Diag fields *on the same Criteria row*. If you do this, you are effectively saying:

Find me cases with:

- *Principal Diag with 'I' as the first character of the Principal Diag code AND*
- *Suburb of 10 or 11 AND*
- *Other Diag01 with either Z8643 or Z720 AND*
- *Other Diag02 with either Z8643 or Z720 AND*
- *Other Diag03 with either Z8643 or Z720 (etc.).*

The data files in the healthcare system that record the diagnoses of inpatient care do not repeat diagnosis codes. Therefore, instead of asking whether the smoker codes are in:

Other Diag01 AND Other Diag02 (and so on)

you need to ask whether the codes are in:

Other Diag01 OR Other Diag02 (and so on).

To achieve this you need to use multiple Criteria rows. If you look closely at the Criteria section of the query design screen, you will see a row which offers the 'or' option, followed by lots of empty rows. Going along each row (including Criteria) represents AND requirements, while rows going down the screen represent OR alternatives (Fig 5.52).

Figure 5.52

Criteria 'or' rows giving additional criteria options

Criteria 'or' rows

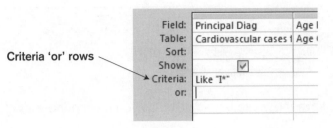

Field:	Principal Diag	Age
Table:	Cardiovascular cases 1	Age
Sort:		
Show:	☑	
Criteria:	Like 'I*'	
or:		

You need to set up a row of criteria for each OR requirement – each row has to find cases that have 'I' starting the Principal Diag code, 10 or 11 as the Suburb, and Z720 or Z8643 in each of the Other Diag fields.

EXERCISE 5.1 CONTINUED

27 Figure 5.53 shows what is needed to set up all the criteria correctly. Still in Design View, copy and paste the different criteria into the boxes as shown.

Field:	Principle Diag	Age Group	Age Description	Age Description	Suburb	Other Diag01	Other Diag02	Other Diag03
Table:	Cardiovascular cases 1	Cardiovascular cases 1	Age Group Codes	Age Group Codes	Cardiovascular cases 1	Cardiovascular cases 1	Cardiovascular cases 1	Cardiovascular ca
Sort:								
Show:	☑	☑	☑	☑	☑	☑	☑	☑
Criteria:	Like "I*"				10 Or 11	"Z720" Or "Z8643"		
or:	Like "I*"				10 Or 11		"Z720" Or "Z8643"	
	Like "I*"				10 Or 11			"Z720" Or "Z8643"
	Like "I*"				10 Or 11			
	Like "I*"				10 Or 11			
	Like "I*"				10 Or 11			

Figure 5.53 Multiple requirement specifications

You will reach a point where there are insufficient lines to allow you to enter the requirements for all of the Other Diag fields. In this case you need to insert rows. Left-click in one of the Criteria 'or' rows, then

❑ in Access 2007, add additional rows using the **Design** ribbon (Fig 5.54)
❑ in Access 2003, go to **Insert ➤ Rows**.

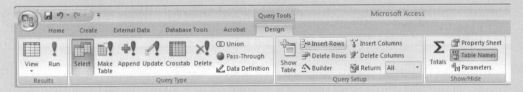

Figure 5.54 Adding rows to the criteria of a query (Access 2007)

28 The end result will show all the cases where smoking has been recorded in any of the Other Diag fields for cases that are circulatory disease and for the local area.

To check that your query has worked, go to the Datasheet View and check the number of entries. In Figure 5.51, there were 72 entries that had a smoking diagnosis; the result of the more extensive specification of criteria gives a higher number as it includes *all* cases where smoking was recorded, not just those where it was recorded in the first 'other diagnosis'. Figure 5.55 (overleaf) shows that 281 of the cardiovascular cases are smokers.

Figure
5.55 All smokers
and ex-smokers

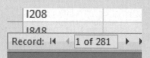

| 1208 |
| 1848 |

Record: |◄ ◄ 1 of 281 ► ►|

It is important to save the query at this point, as you have done a lot of manual work.

Summary
The objectives of this section were to:

- find the smokers (add smoking to the query) – *done*
- record that they are smokers – creating a new field, and filing the field appropriately
- create a new table that holds smoking status
- fill the table with smokers, then add the non-smokers to get a table from which we can produce the required report.

We will now move on to record that these are the smokers and store the results.

5.4.7 Creating a new field in a query

Now that the smokers have been identified, you can 'mark' them by creating a field into which you enter smoking status.

EXERCISE 5.1 CONTINUED

29 In the Design View of the *Smokers/Non Smokers* query saved from question 28, add a field called smoker (Fig 5.56) by typing **Smoker** into an empty Field box.

❑ To structure the Smoker field as a Yes/No field, select that column, right-click and choose **Properties**. For the format of the field, choose Yes/No. This will create a two-option field, displayed as a check box.

❑ Go to Datasheet View – you will be asked to enter a parameter value for the smoker field (Fig 5.56). Type in **Y** to indicate that all the people retrieved are smokers. The result in the Datasheet View is shown in Figure 5.57, which displays a new field on the far right, **Expr1**.

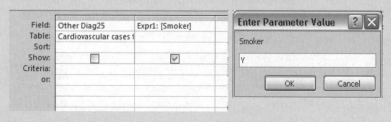

Figure 5.56 Adding a new field and entering a variable

Note that even after saving the query, each time you open it (in Datasheet View) you will be asked to give a value for 'Smoker' – the same thing happens each time you move back into Datasheet View from Design View. This is because you might wish to change the parameter value. If the value is always to be the same you could enter a rule by building a query, but the process used here allows you to use the same field and structure first to indicate the smokers, and then to indicate the non-smokers, by entering the appropriate value in the parameter.

Figure 5.57
Result of field generation (note that here a new column has been added to the right of the suburb column for 'Smoker' (Expr1)

Record ID	Principal Dia	Age Descrip	Suburb	Expr1
736	I619	30-39	11	Y
2408	I800	30-39	11	Y
754	I200	40-49	11	Y
2256	I259	40-49	11	Y
795	I211	40-49	11	Y
407	I209	40-49	10	Y
1904	I848	40-49	11	Y
798	I209	40-49	11	Y
2872	I639	40-49	11	Y
653	I200	50-59	11	Y
965	I200	50-59	10	Y
374	I7023	50-59	10	Y
973	I200	50-59	11	Y
1958	I48	50-59	11	Y
583	I7021	50-59	10	Y
1984	I200	50-59	11	Y
732	I200	50-59	11	Y
699	I200	50-59	11	Y
1293	I200	50-59	11	Y
2848	I839	50-59	11	Y

5.4.8 Creating a new table from a query

Having identified which records belong to smokers, we now need to store these details, including the new field, in a safe place. To do this you can use your query to make a new table into which you put these results.

Types of queries
So far, all the modifications made to the *Smokers/Non Smokers* query have been as a 'Select query'. Queries extract data from tables and can process these results in different ways.

- The **Select query** simply selects information so that it can be displayed and made available for reporting. These queries use display and access processes.
- Queries can also be used to extract and process information, and put the results into a new table where the results are more stable and able to be further processed – this is a **Make-Table query**.

- There are also queries that append data to an existing table – meaning that the entries in the query are added to the end of existing entries in a table. This is the **Append query**.
- The **Update query** updates entries in an existing table with new values, such as updating the fee for all patients receiving a specific service throughout a table.
- The **Delete query** deletes all the selected records from the original source table.
- **Crosstab queries** make analysis of data easier. They calculate the sum, average and count of entries for specified groups of data, and restructure the data to help you find and compare information.

We shall look at how most of these queries work, in the sections below.

Make-Table query

This process uses the query function not just to return values that meet the criteria and calculations established in the query, but also to put the results of the query into a new table.

EXERCISE 5.1 CONTINUED

30 With the existing *Smoker/Non Smokers* query open in **Design View**:
   ❑ in Access 2007, select **Make Table** in the **Query Tools** ribbon
   ❑ in Access 2003, go to **Query ➤ Make-Table Query**.

You will get the dialog box shown in Figure 5.58.

Figure 5.58
Make Table
dialog box

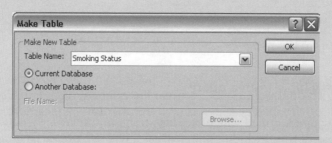

Give the new table a name (e.g. *Smoking Status*), and choose for the new table to be created in your current database. (If you want the table to be put into another database, you must indicate that database's name.) Press **OK**.

You will also notice that the title bar of your query window has changed – Select Query has become Make Table Query (Fig 5.59).

Figure 5.59
Query heading
for the Make
Table Query

Smokers/Non Smokers : Make Table Query

Quick hints

- Saving the Make-Table query will overwrite your original Select query, so if you want to keep the Select query do a Save As.
- You can change the Make-Table query back into a Select query using the same path, but this time choosing 'Select Query' from the menu of options.

Your earlier queries were Select queries (used to select data). You can still check the query process by using the Datasheet View option – this does not create a table, but just lets you see what will be put into the table when you do create it. However, from now on whenever you *open* the query (unless you specifically go to its Design View) it will 'make' the table – replacing what was in the table in the past. You may well get a pop-up window warning you of this.

31 Save the query. When you return to the Query section of the main database window, you will notice that the icon next to the *Smokers/Non Smokers* query is different (Fig 5.60).

Figure 5.60
Query with Make-Table identification icon

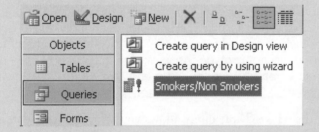

☐ To actually *create* the *Smoking Status* table from the query, you must 'run' the query. To do this you need to open the query straight into Design View (right-click on the query), then press the **Run icon** – an exclamation mark – in the toolbar. Enter the parameter (Y) as before.

The program will create a new table, and ask you to confirm that creation by telling you how many records are to be put into the table (Fig 5.61).

Figure 5.61
New table creation message

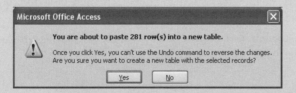

Figure 5.62 (overleaf) shows the new table in the table listing of the main database window. You can now close the query.

Figure 5.62
The new
table created
appears at
the bottom of
the list

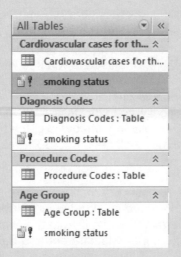

32   Open the new table in Design View. Note that it has design descriptions that
are the same as the fields from the query. The newly created field currently
called Expr1 (a name created automatically by the query process) has brought
in all the records established as needed in the query.

❑   Set the primary key for the new table to **Record ID**. This allows you to
restrict the table to one entry per Record ID. In any table, the primary key
can only occur once (here, only one entry for each individual record number)
– and therefore when you add the content of the Append Query to the table
(the next step), it will not replace those entries that already have a record
number in the new table. Save the table and close it.

Saving the Make-Table query allows you to re-run (re-create) the table at
any time. This is particularly useful if the original data gets updated – you
can simply re-create the table with the new data at any time. This is one of
the benefits of a database. Once the processes are built, they can be used over
and over again. They can also be copied to form the basis of similar queries.

Append query

Our new table currently contains only smokers. The next step is to add the
cases which are not smokers. To do this, we make a copy of the existing Make-
Table query, change this query to append the new table to our existing *Smoking
Status* table rather than replacing it, and then create a table to append.

EXERCISE 5.1 CONTINUED

33   You will need to make a copy of the existing Make-Table query – as the
selection and structure we now want similar to this query, but we don't want
to overwrite the table we have already made. In the main database window,
highlight the query, then right-click and choose **Copy**, then right-click again

and choose **Paste**. If you already have the query open, you can use **Save As** instead. You will be asked to give the query a name (Fig 5.63).

Figure 5.63
Pasting a
copy of the
query with a
new name

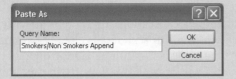

34 Our copied query needs to be altered so that it adds to an existing table rather than making a new table or replacing the old one. Open the copied query in Design View, and change the query type:
   ❑ in Access 2007, go to the **Query Tools** ribbon and select **Append**
   ❑ in Access 2003, go to **Query ➤ Append Query**.

A dialog box will appear, asking for the name of the table to which the appended records are to be sent (Fig 5.64). In this case, the table shown is the one we want (the one created by the previous Make-Table query). Press **OK**.

Figure 5.64
Changing
query type to
append, and
choosing the
destination
table

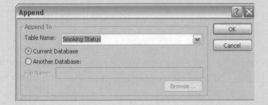

The structure of the query will change automatically. As can be seen in Figure 5.65, there is a new row in the lower section of the Design View, entitled **Append To**. This indicates the names of the fields in the existing *Smoking Status* table in which the result of this query will be put.

Figure 5.65
Append query
table grid

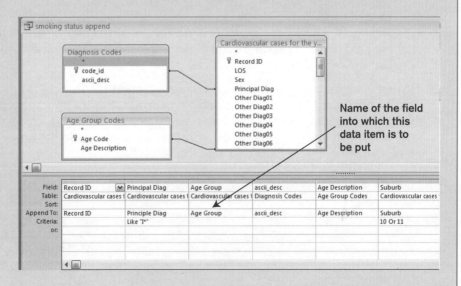

Remember that the objective is to add the records for *non-smokers* to the table recording smoking status. We therefore need to change our query so that the non-smokers are included in the table we create.

There are many ways to achieve this. You *could* create a query that selects only those cases where the value in the Other Diag field is not Z720 and not Z8643, but this is a complex expression and there is an easier way.

The table to which you want to add details already has entries in it, including the Record ID. This is the unique ID for the table entries, meaning that the system will only allow *one* entry in the table with that Record ID. It is possible to use this database fact to advantage in this instance. If the Append query simply selects all relevant cases whether they are smokers or not, and adds *all* of these cases to the newly created table, the system will only accept those entries where the Record ID is not already in the table. As the table currently holds smokers and ex-smokers, the only ones that will be added are the non-smokers.

It is therefore not necessary to include all the Other Diag fields, nor are the criteria to determine smokers needed. Simply delete these fields from the criteria, including the additional rows you had added. There is only one line of criteria necessary – the one that identifies the diagnosis and the suburb. You do not need to have a 'smoking' field as this field already exists in the table to which you are adding data, and will be left blank if you do not give an instruction that will fill it. Figure 5.65 shows the criteria required.

EXERCISE 5.1 CONTINUED

35 To add the records for *non-smokers* to the table recording smoking status, we don't need to change the cardiovascular disease and suburb criteria, but the criterion for the Other Diag fields has to change – we have to delete the restriction to 'smoker'.
- ❒ Left-click in the **Criteria** box under **Other Diag01** and highlight and delete the text in that cell. Then delete the text in all the **or** rows for the rest of the Other Diag fields.
- ❒ Now go to Datasheet View. You will be asked to enter a parameter value for the field 'Expr1'. Leave it blank – we will look at this in a later step. Check that the record count is now 1179.

36 When you are happy with your query, save it and then **Run** the Append query, and confirm the append at the warning message (Fig 5.66). The number of rows is 1179 because the database will try to add all the smokers too, but will not be able to as Record ID already exists in the table, and the database will not let a second entry be recorded with the same ID.

Figure 5.66
Append
confirmation

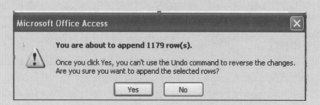

Microsoft Office Access

You are about to append 1179 row(s).

Once you click Yes, you can't use the Undo command to reverse the changes. Are you sure you want to append the selected rows?

[Yes]   [No]

Open the new table to check it: the non-smokers will now have an entry (N or blank) in the Expr1 field.

37 You can improve the table in a couple of ways.
The field name *Expr1* is not meaningful, and should be changed to 'Smoker'. This can be done in either view.
- ❑ In Design View, double-click on the field name and type over it.
- ❑ In Datasheet View, double-click on the column heading and type over it (Fig 5.67).

Also, in Design View, change the Data Type for the Smoker field to 'Yes/No'. This will give you tick boxes.

Figure 5.67
Renamed
field –
Smoker

Record ID ▾	Principal Dia ▾	Age Descrip ▾	Suburb ▾	Smoker
1551	I472	60-69	10	N
1583	I471	60-69	10	N
1534	I471	60-69	11	N
1584	I471	60-69	10	N
1594	I471	60-69	10	N
521	I351	60-69	11	N
1542	I455	60-69	11	N
676	I351	60-69	10	N
1517	I447	60-69	11	N
696	I442	60-69	11	N
1527	I442	60-69	11	N
888	I442	60-69	11	N
215	I429	60-69	11	N

Figure 5.68 shows how the new table should look after step 37 of Exercise 5.1.

Figure 5.68
New table
showing smokers
and non-smokers

⊞ Smoking Status					
Record ID ▾	Principal Dia ▾	ascii_desc ▾	Age Group ▾	Age Descrip ▾	Smoker ▾
8	I842	Internal haem	5	50 - 59	☐
13	I842	Internal haem	5	50 - 59	☐
18	I841	Internal haem	7	70 - 79	☐
19	I839	Varicose veins	5	50 - 59	☐
23	I269	Pulmonary em	7	70 - 79	☐
27	I978	Other postpro	8	80 - 89	☐
29	I849	Unspecified ha	7	70 - 79	☐
39	I269	Pulmonary em	5	50 - 59	☐
40	I842	Internal haem	5	50 - 59	☐
49	I842	Internal haem	6	60 - 69	☐
58	I841	Internal haem	6	60 - 69	☐
61	I839	Varicose veins	7	70 - 79	☐
65	I849	Unspecified ha	6	60 - 69	☐

Record: I◄ ◄ 1 of 1179 ► ►I ►¤ ☒ No Filter   Search

Update query

Suburb names could be added by creating a lookup or reference table as was done with age groups, but in this case there are only two suburbs to be named, so names will be added using Update query to provide an example of this functionality.

Exercise 5.1 continued

38 The first step in adding suburb names is to change the format of the Suburb field from a number to text. Open the table in Design View and update the Data Type from number to text (Fig 5.69). Save the change, and view the result. You will notice that the numbers which were on the right-hand side of the column (as numbers always are) are now on the left-hand side, as text.

Figure 5.69
Data types
required

⊞ Smoking Status	
Field Name	**Data Type**
⚷ Record ID	Number
Principal Diag	Text
Age Group	Number
ascii_desc	Text
Age Description	Text
Suburb	Text
Smoker	Yes/No

39 Create a new query in Design View. This new query is based on the newly created *Smoking Status* table, so add that table to the query (Fig 5.70). Close the dialog box, and place the Suburb field into the query.

Figure 5.70
Choose the
table with the
data to be
updated

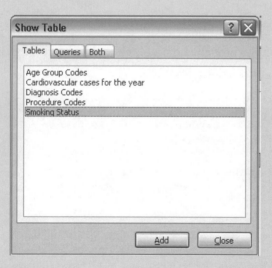

In the Suburb field there are two values, 10 and 11. Suburb 10 is Hightown, while suburb 11 is Central City. We have to change each one separately. First, enter the restriction criteria for suburb 10 (Fig 5.71).

Figure 5.71
Criteria for
selecting
suburb 10

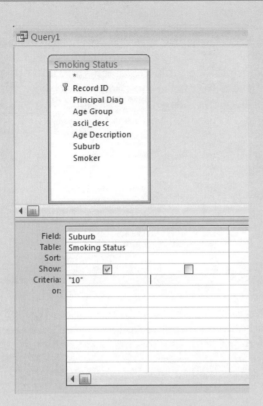

❏ Next, change the query type to Update Query. The details displayed in the table grid rows change, from 'Sort' and 'Show' to 'Update To' (Fig 5.72). Enter the name Hightown in the Update To box; the system will automatically put quotation marks around the text.

Figure 5.72
Update
Query,
showing
'Update To'
row

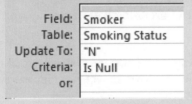

❏ Press the **Run** button. You will be warned that 257 rows will be modified. Because you limited the query to suburb 10, only those rows will be updated. The resulting updates to the *Smoking Status* table is shown in Figure 5.73. Save the table. You do not have to save the Update query.

Figure 5.73 Hightown showing in the modified table

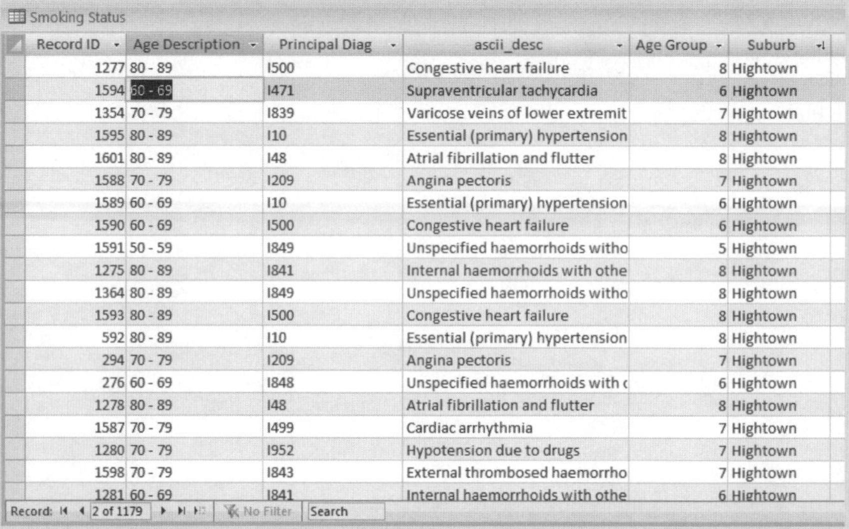
Smoking Status

Record ID	Age Description	Principal Diag	ascii_desc	Age Group	Suburb
1277	80 - 89	I500	Congestive heart failure	8	Hightown
1594	60 - 69	I471	Supraventricular tachycardia	6	Hightown
1354	70 - 79	I839	Varicose veins of lower extremit	7	Hightown
1595	80 - 89	I10	Essential (primary) hypertension	8	Hightown
1601	80 - 89	I48	Atrial fibrillation and flutter	8	Hightown
1588	70 - 79	I209	Angina pectoris	7	Hightown
1589	60 - 69	I10	Essential (primary) hypertension	6	Hightown
1590	60 - 69	I500	Congestive heart failure	6	Hightown
1591	50 - 59	I849	Unspecified haemorrhoids witho	5	Hightown
1275	80 - 89	I841	Internal haemorrhoids with othe	8	Hightown
1364	80 - 89	I849	Unspecified haemorrhoids witho	8	Hightown
1593	80 - 89	I500	Congestive heart failure	8	Hightown
592	80 - 89	I10	Essential (primary) hypertension	8	Hightown
294	70 - 79	I209	Angina pectoris	7	Hightown
276	60 - 69	I848	Unspecified haemorrhoids with c	6	Hightown
1278	80 - 89	I48	Atrial fibrillation and flutter	8	Hightown
1587	70 - 79	I499	Cardiac arrhythmia	7	Hightown
1280	70 - 79	I952	Hypotension due to drugs	7	Hightown
1598	70 - 79	I843	External thrombosed haemorrho	7	Hightown
1281	60 - 69	I841	Internal haemorrhoids with othe	6	Hightown

Record: 2 of 1179 No Filter Search

40 An alternative method is to open the *Smoking Status* table in Datasheet View, select the Suburb field and use the **Replace** option to change the text, similar to how this is done in Word or Excel. Use this method to change suburb 11 to Central City.

5.4.9 Adding simple calculations to queries

Although the Report generator (see section 5.5) can prepare calculations, there is more flexibility if the calculations are prepared in a query – the results of the calculations are available for inclusion in reports *as well as* the original source data.

We will use the example of grouping data. To recap, the Exercise 5.1 question asks for:

> the difference in prevalence of disease and age group of the people represented in this file according to whether they are smokers or not.

Thus, the calculation required is to *group* the cases according to age group, smoker/non-smoker status and prevalence of disease, and identify how many cases there are in each of these groups.

Exercise 5.1 continued

41 Create a new query in Design View, add the table *Smoking Status*, and place the fields Age Description, ascii_desc and Smoker into the query design grid (Fig 5.74).

Figure 5.74
Fields required
for grouping
query

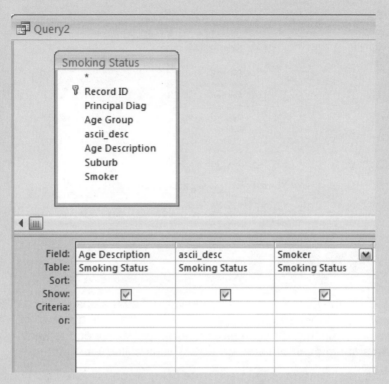

To perform the grouping calculation, we use the **Total** function. This appears as an icon with the summation sign ∑, in the **Query Tools** ribbon (Access 2007) or the toolbar (Access 2003). See Figure 5.75.

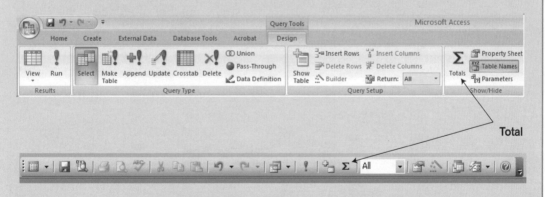

Total

Figure 5.75 Total button in (top) Access 2007 and (bottom) Access 2003

This will add a **Total** row to the design grid in your query (Fig 5.76, overleaf).

Figure 5.76
Total line appears
in query when the
Total icon is
pressed

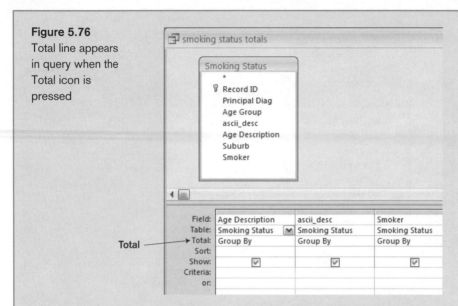

Total

Now go to the Datasheet View – you will notice that instead of 1179 records (rows) in the table, there are now only 361. This is because there now is only one row for each group of similar record. You now need to know *how many* records are in each of these groups. This is called a **count**.

❏ The count needs to be a separate field, so go back to Datasheet View and place the Smoker field into a second column in the design grid (so 'Smoker' will appear twice).

❏ In this second Smoker column, left-click on the words **Group By** and then use the look-up arrow (the down-arrow that appear on the right of the box) to select **Count** (Fig 5.77). This will count the number of entries in the grouped row.

Figure 5.77
Choosing a
'Group By'
function from the
list available

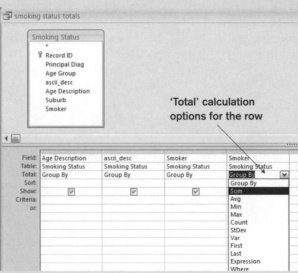

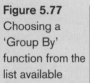

□ Go back to Datasheet View, and look at the results to check that they seem appropriate (Fig 5.78). Save the query as *Smoking status totals for report.*

Figure 5.78
Result of
count in
query

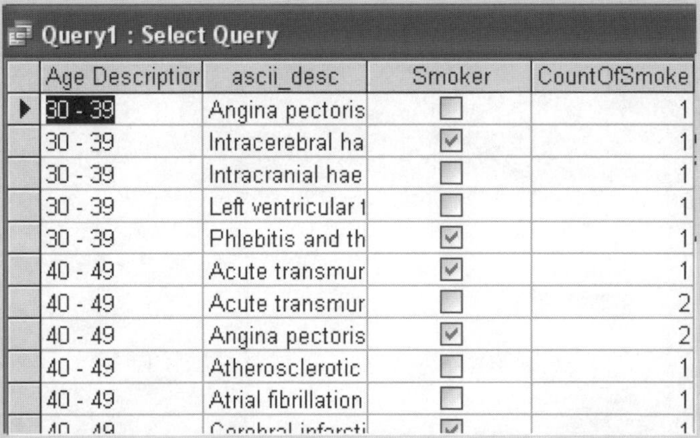

Query1 : Select Query

Age Description	ascii_desc	Smoker	CountOfSmoke
▶ 30 - 39	Angina pectoris	☐	1
30 - 39	Intracerebral ha	☑	1
30 - 39	Intracranial hae	☐	1
30 - 39	Left ventricular f	☐	1
30 - 39	Phlebitis and th	☑	1
40 - 49	Acute transmur	☑	1
40 - 49	Acute transmur	☐	2
40 - 49	Angina pectoris	☑	2
40 - 49	Atherosclerotic	☐	1
40 - 49	Atrial fibrillation	☐	1
40 - 49	Cerebral infarcti	☑	1

You now have all the components needed to move on to reporting.

5.5 Producing reports

In this section you will produce reports with the data you have prepared so far in Exercise 5.1.

You will need to identify *what* report you are trying to produce. In Exercise 5.1, we want to produce a report of cases of people admitted to hospital with cardiovascular conditions; the report also needs to indicate whether they are smokers or not, and the age group into which they fall.

Before you begin a report, you should know which query or table will form the basis of your report. It is also important to have a clear vision of how you would like the report to look. You must understand which fields you want to see, what headings, any statistics, etc.

For Exercise 5.1, our report will be based on the query *Smoking Status Report Totals*, and it will include smoking status, age and diagnosis data. Headings will be used for smoking status and age group.

5.5.1 Report Wizard

Access provides a Report Wizard, a series of dialog boxes that guide you through developing the report content, look and feel.

EXERCISE 5.1 CONTINUED

42 In the main database window, go to the **Reports** section (Fig 5.79). Any existing will be listed here (there are currently none).

Figure 5.79
Reports
section of
main
database
window in
Access 2003

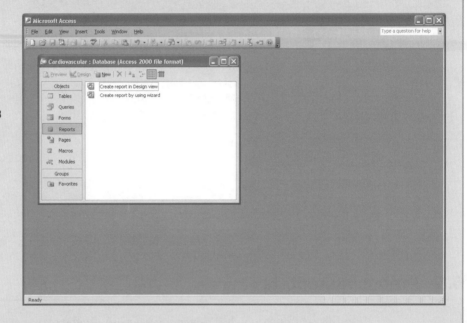

☐ In Access 2007, go to **Create ➤ Reports ➤ Report Wizard**.
☐ In Access 2003, choose **Create report by using wizard** from the list.

When the Report Wizard window first opens, it displays details for the first table on the list alphabetically – you often need to change this selection (Figure 5.80).

Figure 5.80
Initial window
of Report
Wizard,
showing table
that has been
actively
selected

Selecting data for reporting

Note from Figure 5.80 that you can select fields for the report from more than one table or query. In our simple example, all the data we want is in the one query.

EXERCISE 5.1 *CONTINUED*

43 Left-click on the down-arrow to the right of the 'Tables/Queries' box to get a list of all tables and Select Queries that exist for the database (Fig 5.81). The tables and queries are presented in alphabetical order. Select **Query: Smoking status totals for report**. This is the grouped query we created in step 41 of Exercise 5.1.

Figure 5.81
Table/Query
selection

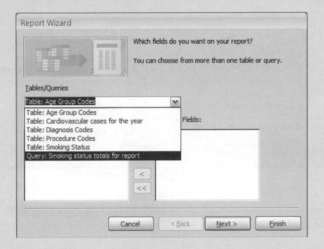

When you make this selection, the **Available Fields** list will become populated with the names of all the fields in the selected table (Fig 5.82).

Figure 5.82
Report
Wizard
showing
available
fields

Next, you need to select the fields to be included in the report, in the order you wish them to appear on the report.

- ❒ Select by double-clicking on an individual field, or by highlighting the field and using the single right-arrow to move the item to the right-hand box (where it will be included in the report). The double arrows move *all* the fields to the right-hand box. Once a field is selected (appears in the right-hand box), the left-arrows will become active so that you can move items back to the left-hand box (i.e. de-select them).
- ❒ Select all the fields in *Query: Smoking status totals for report*, in the order shown in Figure 5.83. Press **Next**.

Figure 5.83
Selected data items for the report

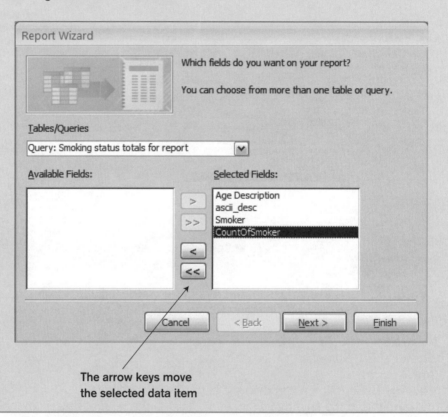

The arrow keys move the selected data item

Grouping and sorting

The Report Wizard offers assistance with the creation of headings or statistical groups in a report. Groups are used for modifying the layout of the report, developing headings, and giving the option to provide statistics for groups of information.

Figure 5.84
Report Wizard
Step 2: grouping

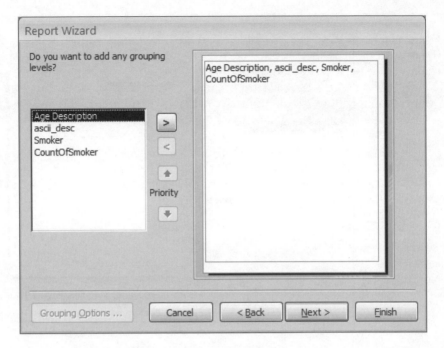

Figure 5.84 shows the grouping screen. The way you group the information will be dependent upon the way you need to view the information in the final report. For example:

- If you were interested in the variations of age and smoking status for individual diseases, you would sort by disease (as in our example).
- If you were more interested in the disease and smoking status relationships within age groups, you would sort by different age groups.

The report will group the information according to your selection and the groups will be presented sorted in alphabetical order.

EXERCISE 5.1 CONTINUED

44 Age Description holds the details of the age group to which a person belongs, and this is the field by which we will group the information. This choice is based on the need to understand the different impact of smoking on people in different age groups.
  ❏ Create the group by highlighting **Age Description** on the left and clicking the arrow button (or double-clicking on **Age Description**).

When a group is selected it is displayed as in Figure 5.85, which shows the layout that will be produced by the group choice. If you have more than one group, you can change the priority up and down, i.e. changing the hierarchy of the groups and thus changing the layout.

Figure 5.85
Group
choices

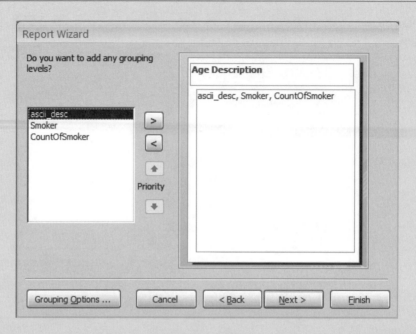

Once a grouping choice is made, the **Grouping Options** button is also activated. This allows you to group on part of a field. For example, if you were using ICD10 codes you could group on the first three characters; this would group E10.10 with E10.20 as they have the same first three digits. That is not necessary in this case.

45 After you have set up the group as in Figure 5.85, press **Next**. You will be offered options for sorting data in the report (Fig 5.86).

Figure 5.86
Sorting and
summary/
statistical
information

Report Wizard

What sort order and summary information do you want for detail records?

You can sort records by up to four fields, in either ascending or descending order.

1 [▾] Ascending
2 [▾] Ascending
3 [▾] Ascending
4 [▾] Ascending

Summary Options ...

Cancel   < Back   Next >   Finish

In our example, the system will automatically sort by the age description, as it sorts first by fields that are used for grouping. We can add more detailed sorting within the group through the indication of a sort sequence. Choose the **ascii_desc** field as the sort sequence.

Report statistics

The report would also be suitable for analysis if you include statistics that list totals for each group. If your selected fields include numerical data, the Report Wizard will activate the Summary Options button, which offers some statistical calculations. In our case, the Count of Smoker field will trigger this option.

When statistics are requested, Access will automatically count the number of records in the group – provided that we ask for some statistics, we don't have to tell Access to count. Figure 5.87 lists the fields available in our query for statistical analysis, and offers some simple statistics. We can do any of summary (total), average, minimum and maximum calculations for each Smoker or Count of Smoker field.

EXERCISE 5.1 CONTINUED

46 Press **Summary Options** in the window shown in Figure 5.86, to get the Summary Options window in Figure 5.87.

Figure 5.87
Statistics/
Summary
information
selection

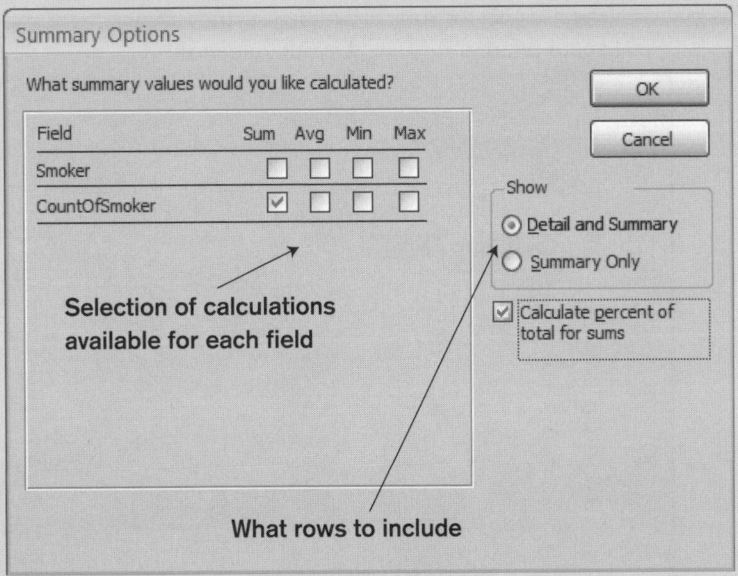

❐ Choose to **Sum** the Count of Smoker field.

❐ You are also able to select whether you want to see a line for every record in your table/query or only the totals: in the **Show** section, choosing 'Summary Only' will give you totals without detailed records. Although this exercise does not ask us to show individual entries, the query we are using contains already summarised data. This means that we need each individual row in this query to appear in the report. Choose **Detail and Summary** in the **Show** section.

❐ Exercise 5.1 requires some way of being able to *compare* the different rates in the community. This can be done most simply using a percentage, as percentages and (other forms of rates) allow comparison between different groups. Choose **Calculate percent of total for sums**.

❐ When you have made all your selections, press **OK**. This will return you to the previous screen of the Report Wizard, where you could choose how to sort the records. Press **Next**.

Layout selection

Access offers a range of layouts for your data. These can be chosen using the layout screen of the Report Wizard (Fig 5.88). There are three main elements. The **Layout** section is where you choose the general look of where the fields will be positioned; as you click on different option, the layout picture will change to reflect this. The **Orientation** section is where you choose the paper/screen format, and there is a check box for selecting whether you want to adjust your display of field widths so that all fields fit on one page.

Figure 5.88
Report Wizard
layout screen

Layout picture   **Layout selection**   **Orientation**

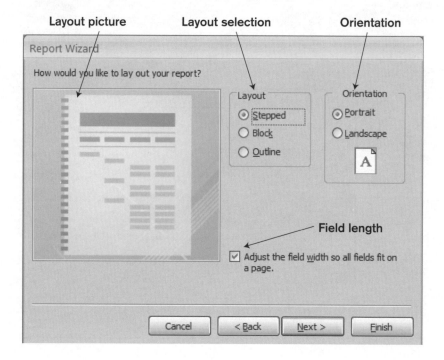

47 When you have made your choices in the layout screen of the Report Wizard (and it is recommended that you try a few to see what you like), press **Next**. Preview the different styles available to select the overall look you prefer (Fig 5.89). Press **Next**.

Figure 5.89
Selection of overall look or style

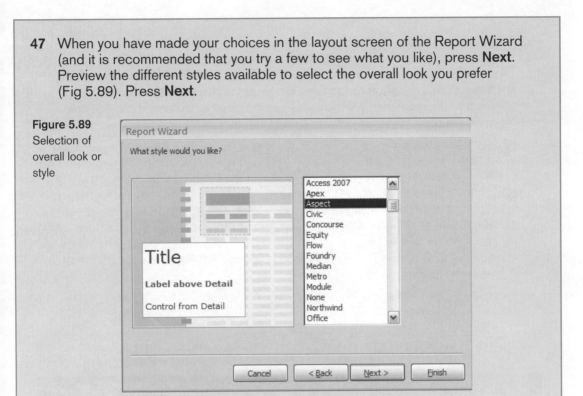

Saving and previewing the report

The next step is to save your report under an appropriate name. If you don't choose a name yourself, Access will default to the name of the query or table upon which you have based your report – see Figure 5.90.

Figure 5.90
Giving the report a name

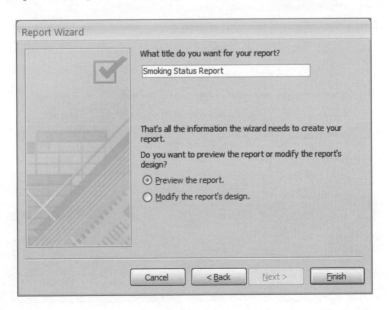

48 Type in a suitable name for your report, such as *Smoking Status Report*. You are then given the option to preview the report. Always do this, because if something has gone badly wrong you can go back to correct it before your report is finalised.

Figure 5.91 shows a preview of the query results. It shows that (for example) in the age group 30–39 there was one person who was a non-smoker who had the diagnosis angina pectoris; lower down, it also shows that in the 40–49 age group there were three people with the diagnosis acute transmural myocardial infarction of the interior wall, of which one was a smoker and two non-smokers.

❏ When you are happy with the result, press **Finish**. Close the print preview of the report – this will return you to the main database window, where you will now be able to see this Report listed (use the left-hand navigation panel to view the listings).

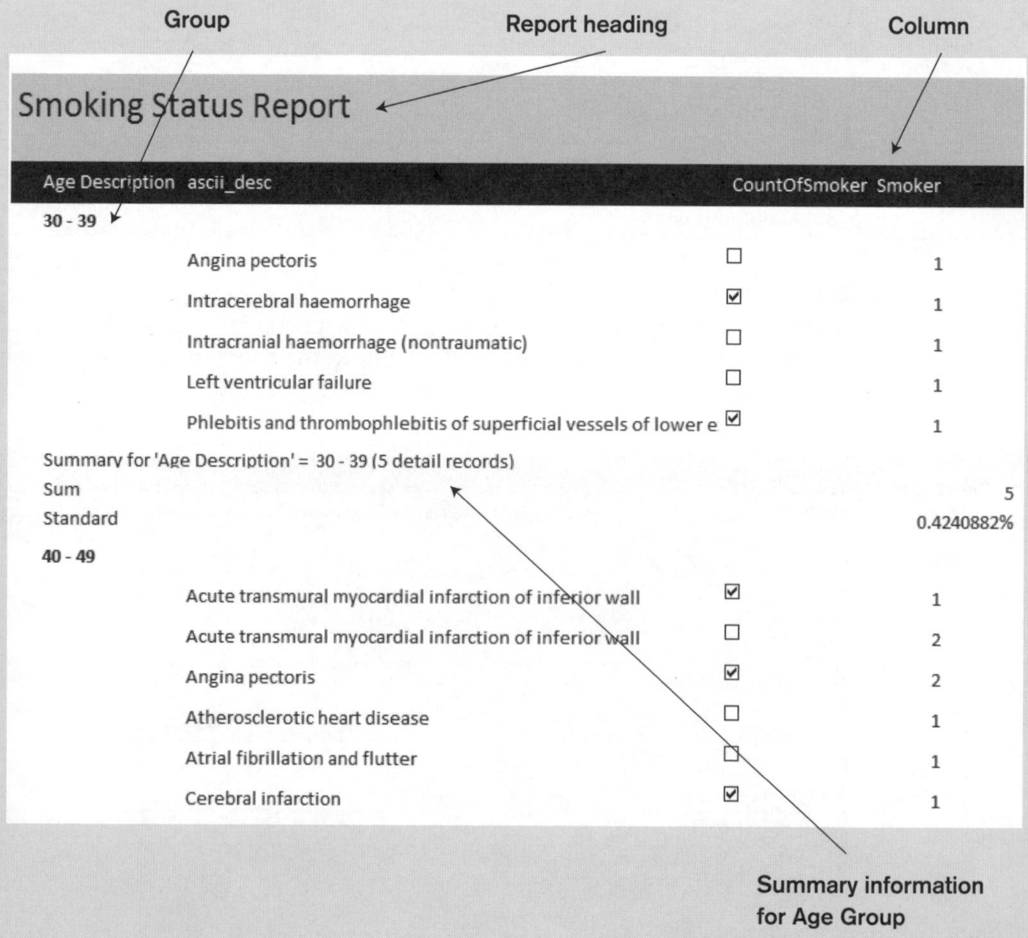

Group   Report heading   Column

Smoking Status Report

Age Description ascii_desc		CountOfSmoker	Smoker
30 - 39			
	Angina pectoris	☐	1
	Intracerebral haemorrhage	☑	1
	Intracranial haemorrhage (nontraumatic)	☐	1
	Left ventricular failure	☐	1
	Phlebitis and thrombophlebitis of superficial vessels of lower e	☑	1
Summary for 'Age Description' = 30 - 39 (5 detail records)			
Sum			5
Standard			0.4240882%
40 - 49			
	Acute transmural myocardial infarction of inferior wall	☑	1
	Acute transmural myocardial infarction of inferior wall	☐	2
	Angina pectoris	☑	2
	Atherosclerotic heart disease	☐	1
	Atrial fibrillation and flutter	☐	1
	Cerebral infarction	☑	1

Summary information for Age Group

Figure 5.91 Report preview

5.5.2 Changing a report in Design View

The look of our report (as shown in Fig 5.91) could be improved. Consider some of the changes below and how they could be achieved:

- Put capitals in the heading.
- Change the column headings so that they make more sense (e.g. 'ascii_desc' would be better called 'Diagnosis'. Also, the column heading for 'CountOfSmoker' could be changed to 'Number'.
- Make the diagnosis display (currently under the 'ascii_desc' header) longer so that it shows the whole text. Also, make the area showing percentage larger so that the whole number shows.
- Make the statistical section look cleaner.

Changes to reports are made in Design View, in the same way that changes to queries or tables are made in Design View.

EXERCISE 5.1 CONTINUED

49 Open your smoking status report in Design View. You will get something similar to Figure 5.92.

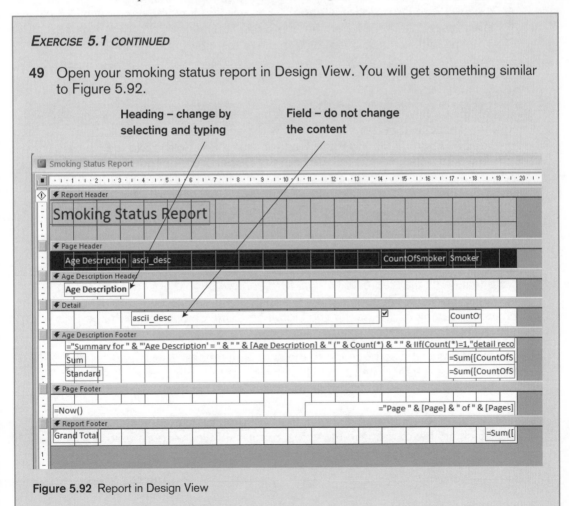

Figure 5.92 Report in Design View

Most changes are made in a manner similar to that in a Microsoft Word document. Each time you try something, click on **Print Preview** to check how it looks, then return to **Design View** to alter.

❑ Go to the **Page Header** and select this heading **ascii_desc**. Now type in the new heading **Diagnosis**. In a similar way, change the page headings **Age Description** to **Age Group**, and **CountOfSmoker** to **Number**.

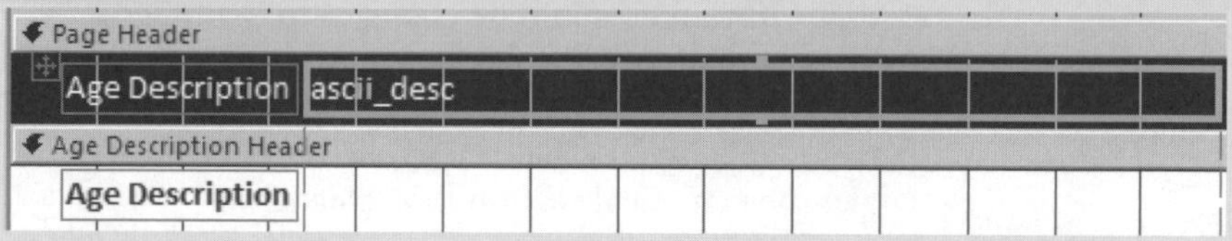

Figure 5.93
Selecting a
heading in
Design View
of the report

❑ You can also use the selection handles to change the item's shape. Try reducing the size of the box that the Age Description fits in (you will find in the area **Age Description Header**). You will find that you can now make the **Diagnosis** column wider so that more text fits in.

❑ You can left-click and drag items to move them on the page too.

Quick hint

To keep things tidy, select two objects at once and move or enlarge them together. This way they will stay aligned with each other. For example, left-click on **Diagnosis** in the **Page Header** area. Now hold down the **Shift** key, and left-click on **ascii_desc** in the **Detail** area. Let go of both Shift and your mouse button; both boxes should now have little black handles on. Hover over the left-hand side of one of the boxes until you get a left-right double-headed arrow. Left-click on this and drag the boxes out to the left to enlarge them.

Note that items that represent *actual field content* should not have their contents modified, although their size and position can be changed. If you change the name of the field in the **Detail** area, the computer won't know which field to present.

50 Modifications can also be made to the summary details. This is particularly useful for the summary heading, which does not look attractive in the form created by the report. It also contains field names that may need to be made more explicit.

For example, Figure 5.94 shows the background instructions that produce the Summary heading line in the actual report, shown in Figure 5.95.

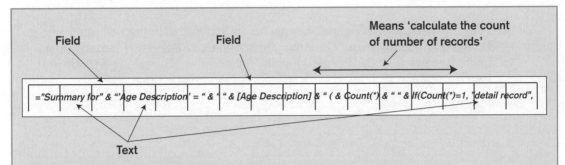

Figure 5.94 Summary heading line instructions generated in initial report

Figure 5.95
Summary heading
line as it appears
in the report

Summary for 'Age Description' = 30 - 39 (5 detail records)

This complex instruction could be made clearer by changing the title 'Age Description' to 'Age Group' – as this is the new column heading we have typed the report's layout. (We could also remove the single quote marks.)

The number of 'detail records' comes from the number of lines (records) represented in this group. In this example this is not particularly useful, and that part of the text could be removed.

❐ Make changes to the summary heading line to get the result shown in Figure 5.96.

Figure 5.96
Improved design for
summary heading line

="Summary for " & "Age Group = " & " " & [Age Description]

The result of this change is a summary heading line as shown in Figure 5.97.

Figure 5.97
Changed summary
heading line, in
preview of report

Summary for Age Group = 30 – 39

51 Having changed the heading, the look of the rest of the summary should be considered. The look and readability of the summary line could be improved by making it larger.

❐ Select the whole line (by clicking on the area to get the box with handles on).

❐ Once the box and handles appears, you will also see a formatting toolbar appear near the top of the main Access window. Here you can modify the font in the same way you would in Word.

❏ Change the font to 10pt and remove the italics. Still with the box highlighted, use your keyboard arrows to move the summary heading line closer to the count to make it easier to read. Finally, change the subheading **Standard** to **Percentage**.

Your report's Design View should now look similar to Figure 5.98.

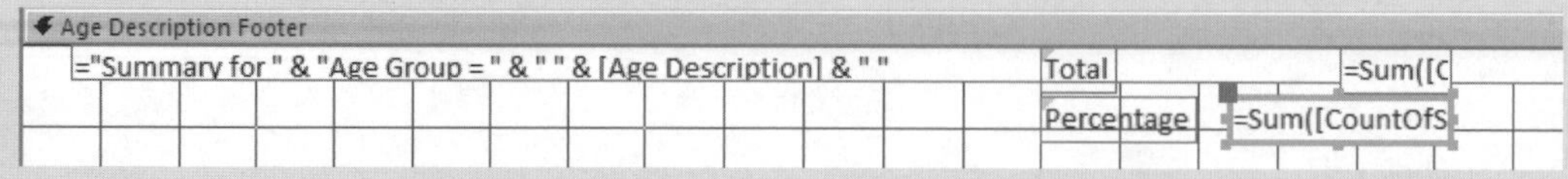

◆ Age Description Footer

="Summary for " & "Age Group = " & " " & [Age Description] & " "								Total		=Sum([C
								Percentage	=Sum([CountOfS	

Figure 5.98 Age Description Footer showing modifications

Preview your report – it should look something like Figure 5.99.

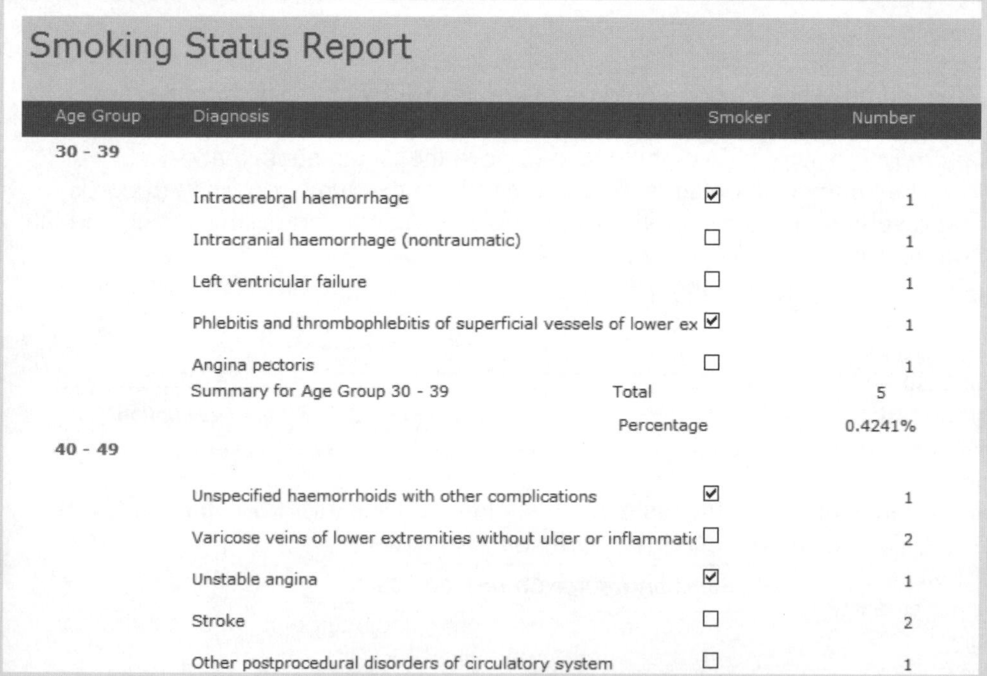

Smoking Status Report

Age Group	Diagnosis	Smoker	Number
30 - 39			
	Intracerebral haemorrhage	☑	1
	Intracranial haemorrhage (nontraumatic)	☐	1
	Left ventricular failure	☐	1
	Phlebitis and thrombophlebitis of superficial vessels of lower ex	☑	1
	Angina pectoris	☐	1
	Summary for Age Group 30 - 39 Total		5
	Percentage		0.4241%
40 - 49			
	Unspecified haemorrhoids with other complications	☑	1
	Varicose veins of lower extremities without ulcer or inflammatic	☐	2
	Unstable angina	☑	1
	Stroke	☐	2
	Other postprocedural disorders of circulatory system	☐	1

Figure 5.99 Report sample showing modified summary layout and heading

Quick hint

Access defaults to two decimal places, so you will only need to do the following if you wish to display more or fewer than this.

52 There are still two elements that could be improved. First, the percentage statistic could be expressed to only one decimal place; second, the diagnosis description for 'Phlebitis and thrombophlebitis of superficial . . .' has been truncated.

To change the details of how a field is displayed, you need to change the properties of that field.

- In Design View, select the line that does the percentage calculation and open the Properties box by right-clicking and selecting **Properties**.
- This dialog box (Fig 5.100) gives details of the format of the data and rules for the data itself. Go to the **All** tab. Left-click in the box to the right of **Decimal Places**, and a down-arrow will appear, giving you a drop-down list of options. Choose **1** decimal place. Close the dialog box.

Figure 5.100
Text Box
properties dialog
box showing all
details

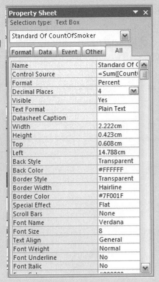

Property Sheet	▼ ×
Selection type: Text Box	
Standard Of CountOfSmoker	⌄

Format	Data	Event	Other	All

Name	Standard Of C
Control Source	=Sum([Count]
Format	Percent
Decimal Places	4
Visible	Yes
Text Format	Plain Text
Datasheet Caption	
Width	2.222cm
Height	0.423cm
Top	0.608cm
Left	14.788cm
Back Style	Transparent
Back Color	#FFFFFF
Border Style	Transparent
Border Width	Hairline
Border Color	#7F001F
Special Effect	Flat
Scroll Bars	None
Font Name	Verdana
Font Size	8
Text Align	General
Font Weight	Normal
Font Underline	No
Font Italic	No

Quick hint

The data formats you have available are summarised below. Clicking on the drop-down list for Format in the Format tab brings up a list with an example shown on the right of each. You may need to make the Properties box wider or longer to be able to see them.

- A selection of date and time formats
- General Number – no format other than the decimal point, with the number of decimal places required mathematically
- Currency – $ sign
- Euro – currency with the Euro symbol
- Fixed – fixed format with the number of decimal places you specify
- Standard – similar to Fixed but has a comma to indicate thousands
- Percent – figure represented as a percentage and using the % symbol
- Scientific – using scientific notation
- True/False
- Yes/No
- On/Off

53 The last thing to fix is that Diagnosis descriptions don't always show fully. This is also done by changing the properties of the field: changing the option 'Can Grow' to 'Yes'. This causes textual data items that don't fit into the space you have to wrap around, using as many lines as needed to display the content of the field.

❑ Select the field **ascii_desc** in the **Detail** section of Design View, and bring up the properties dialog box. Under the **Format** tab, change **Can Grow** to **Yes**. Close the box, and preview your report.

The final report should be similar to Figure 5.101, with the diagnosis text able to cover multiple lines and the percentage shown with one decimal place.

Figure 5.101
Last page of
final report,
showing
Grand Total

Occlusion and stenosis of carotid artery	☐	1	
Stroke	☑	1	
Supraventricular tachycardia	☐	1	
Internal haemorrhoids with other complications	☐	1	
Angina pectoris	☐	2	
Other intracerebral haemorrhage	☑	1	
Hypotension	☐	1	
Embolism and thrombosis of arteries of lower extremities	☐	1	
Congestive heart failure	☐	4	
Congestive heart failure	☑	1	
Cerebral infarction	☐	1	
Atherosclerosis of arteries of extremities	☐	1	
Acute transmural myocardial infarction of inferior wall	☑	1	
Unspecified haemorrhoids with other complications	☐	3	
Atherosclerosis of arteries of extremities with ulceration	☐	1	
Summary for Age Group 90 and over	Total		18
	Percentage		2.0%
Grand Total			**1179**

5.6 Extracting data into other media

The Microsoft Office suite provides facilities for transferring report results to other Office applications.

- In Access 2007, these are found under **External Data ➤ Export** (Fig 5.102).
- In Access 2003, look for the OfficeLinks icon in the toolbar (or go to **Tools ➤ Office Links**) when you have a report open (Fig 5.103). Note that the OfficeLinks icon changes depending on which option is active.

The most common export mechanisms are:

- Excel (which opens the data in the report in a spreadsheet for you to action further, such as graphics).

- Sharepoint – offers the facility to share information through the Internet or Intranet. This is not described in detail here, as it is not a standard part of Microsoft Office functionality.
- Word (which opens the report in a Word file, allowing you to modify the look of the document).

Some of the more useful export functions for the report results are described below.

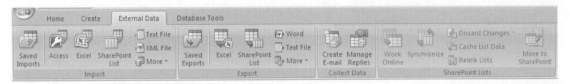

Figure 5.102 External Data ribbon in Access 2007

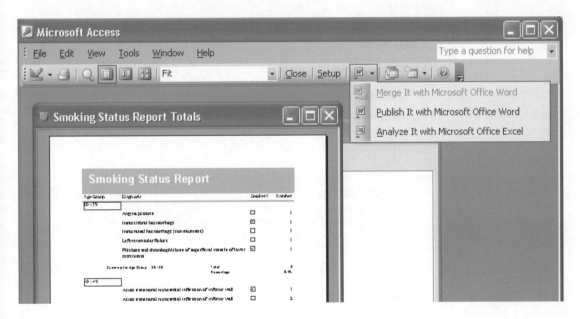

Figure 5.103 OfficeLinks Toolbar icon in Access 2003

Merge with Microsoft Office Word

An example of the use of this option is a report of address details that need to be put into a Word file for printing envelopes. This option will only be active where the data provided is suited to this activity (in our Exercise 5.1 example, it is not).

Publish with Microsoft Office Word

Figure 5.104 shows the report from Exercise 5.1 as it looks when exported into Word; some of the formatting is lost. When this option is chosen, Access opens a Word document and creates a version of the report that is suited to Word.

Smoking Status Report			
Age Group	Diagnosis	Smoker	Number
30–39	Angina pectoris	o	1
	Intracerebral haemorrhage	o	1
	Intracranial haemorrhage (nontraumatic)	o	1
	Left ventricular failure	o	1
	Phlebitis and thrombophlebitis of superficial vessels of lower extremities	o	1
Summary for 'Age Group' = 30–39		Total	5
		Percentage	0.4%
40–49			
	Acute transmural myocardial infarction of inferior wall	o	1
	Acute transmural myocardial infarction of inferior wall	o	2
	Angina pectoris	o	2
	Atherosclerotic heart disease	o	1
	Atrial fibrillation and flutter	o	1
	Cerebral infarction	o	1

Figure 5.104 Example of a report extracted to Microsoft Word

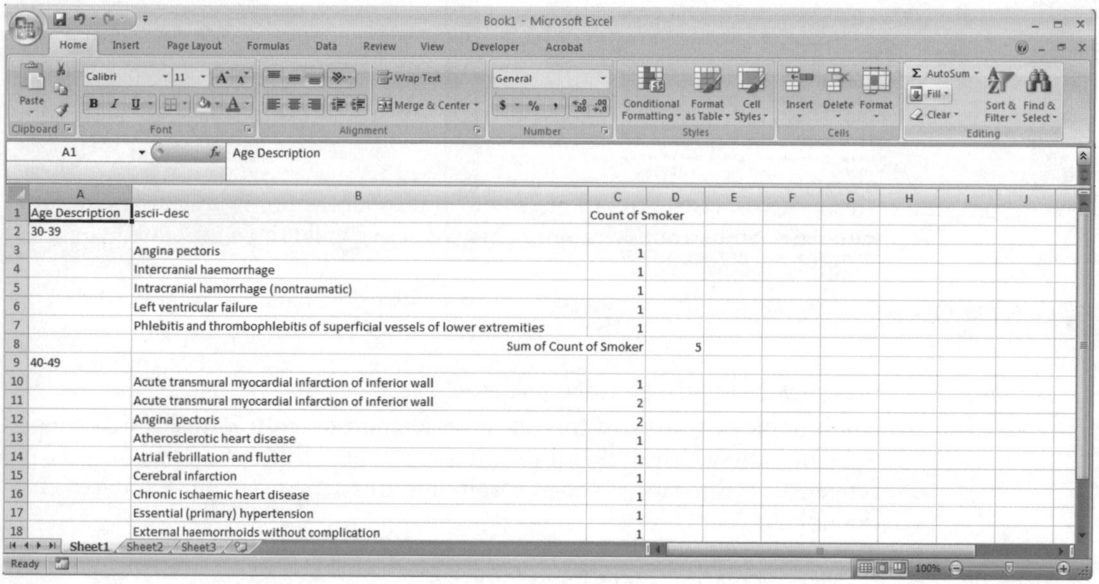

Figure 5.105 Report exported to Excel

Analyse with Microsoft Office Excel

When this option is chosen, Access will automatically open an Excel file, and will insert the report's structure and data into a worksheet (Fig 5.105).

The format of the report does note directly translate between Access and Excel in Office – note that the tick boxes are lost and the data is no longer clear. This happens because the tick box field type is difficult for Excel to automatically handle. If you are likely to want to export a report to Excel, you should consider issues like this when designing your report.

5.7   Developing and creating databases

In earlier sections, we went through the steps of using an existing database. Now we will move on to developing and creating databases for collecting information for specific purposes.

It is quite common that computer services staff do not encourage people in their organisations to develop databases in the work environment. This is largely because the design of such databases is often poor, and either not documented or poorly documented. This means that they are very difficult to maintain or update when the person who created them changes job or leaves the organisation and others have to take the databases over.

When you create a database, you apply the same concepts as when you create a new filing or form system. You must understand both how you intend to capture the information and how you will need to retrieve the information – so that you can design a system which makes this collection and reporting as simple as possible.

The following sections of this book aim to give you the skills to develop a sound database that could be easily maintained by others.
As in the first part of this chapter, we will work through an exercise in the text, and then you should complete similar tasks on a second practice exercise on your own. These exercises assume that you have already worked through Exercises 5.1 and 5.2 so are comfortable finding your way around a database. Steps and techniques covered above will not be explained again in detail in the following sections.

The exercise tasks require you to consider how data will be collected in addition to the possibility of using data that is already on file. Both exercises involve looking at a simple data collection process where we already have a patient index. This is equivalent to saying that we already have patient details, but we now need to collect, store and retrieve information about a specific patient service.

Details of the exercises are given below.

Exercise 5.3

- This exercise requires you to build a database of your own to collect data about patients waiting for treatment.
- The database must be established to handle the organisation's three waiting lists. It is to indicate which waiting lists patients are put on (the

waiting list specifications will be provided below); the urgency of each patient on the waiting lists; and the current status of each patient on the waiting lists (only those patients who have not been allocated a treatment time should be shown on the lists).

- A complete solution is provided in the database called *WaitingList.mdb*.

Exercise 5.4 *(SELF-STUDY)*

- This self-directed exercise aims to give you practice in developing your own database to collect and analyse information.
- In this case you are to develop a data collection system for people attending a community centre so that these patients can be sent follow-up letters to remind them of the need for a pap smear.
- A complete solution is provided on the CD for you to check your progress against. The files are *Recalls.mdb*, *Recall letter template.doc* and *Recall letter result.doc*.

Both exercises use fictitious patient details files. These files are provided as databases on the CD and should be copied to your working directory before you begin the exercises. The file for Exercise 5.3 is *patients.mbd* and that for Exercise 5.4 is *patients for recalls.mdb*.

5.8   Collecting data

The first step is to determine what data needs to be collected, and whether that existing data can be used.

5.8.1   Linking to existing data collections

Where data is already collected, it is good practice to 're-use' it rather than collect it again. In Exercise 5.3 we will use data from the existing data collection called *patients.mdb* provided on the CD.

Before we can link to a data collection, we need to have:

- created a new database to place the data in
- put a copy of the existing data collection into a directory that will always have the same filing relationship to the new database (in the same folder/ directory is good).

In the 'real world' you would be able to access the existing data without having to make a copy or move it. However, for the purposes of the exercises it is easier if you put a copy of the existing data collection onto the device where you are storing your database.

Exercise 5.3

1 Set up a suitable folder/directory for the new database, and copy the database *patients.mdb* into it from the CD.

2 Start up Access and create a new (blank) database, saving it into the same directory under the name *WaitingList.mdb*.

3 Linking to a database involves accessing data that is actually held in a different database, without holding that data in your *own* database. You need to have the new *WaitingList.mdb* database open (it doesn't matter which of the Tables, Queries, Reports or Forms sections is visible). Then:
   ❏ in Access 2007, go to **External Data ➤ Access**
   ❏ in Access 2003, go to **File ➤ Get External Data ➤ Link Tables**.

Figure 5.106 shows the Link dialog box that will come up.

Figure 5.106
Link dialog
box

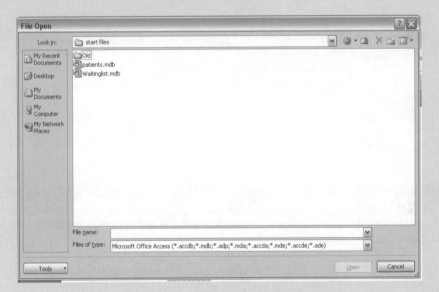

   ❏ Choose to **Link** the *patients.mdb* database. You will then get the Link Tables dialog box, which lists the names of the tables in the database (Fig 5.107). You may choose to link to one or more of these.
   ❏ To provide the information we have been asked for, we only need information from the Patient Details table. Select that table and press **OK**.

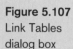

Figure 5.107
Link Tables
dialog box

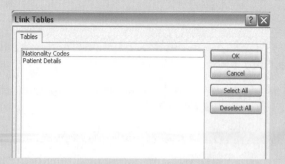

When you select a table to link to, your display returns to the tables section of the main *WaitingList.mdb* database screen, and a new table will now be displayed (Fig 5.108). The small arrow next to the table name indicates that it is a 'virtual' entry in the database – i.e. it is a *link*; the data are not really contained inside *WaitingList.mdb*.

Figure 5.108
Tables
section of
main
database
showing
linked *Patient
Details* table

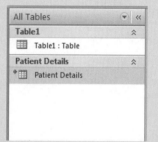

Although the structure and content of the data in the linked table can be seen in Design View from within the *WaitingList.mdb* database, you are not able to modify its structure because it is a linked table. Figure 5.109 shows the structure of the Patient Details table.

Figure 5.109
Patient
Details table
in Design
View

Field Name	Data Type
patient id	AutoNumber
Patient UR number	Text
surname	Text
given name	Text
title	Text
Suffix	Text
date of birth	Date/Time
gender	Text
Nationality Code	Text

5.8.2 Deciding what data to collect

Considering the information available in the Patient Details table, what additional data items are needed for our *WaitingList.mdb* database?

When a patient requires a service of the organisation and there are insufficient resources to meet that need immediately, the person is put onto a waiting list. A person may be on more than one waiting list at any given time. The organisation has requested that a database be developed that allows you to record the details of when the patient was put onto a waiting list, their urgency and current status (are they still waiting?). When the person receives an admission appointment, they are no longer considered to be waiting.

To build such a system, it is important first to understand what information must be collected in order to manage the waiting list system (this is not dissimilar to thinking about a data collection form – and what information you need to collect in a manual system). It is also important to understand how the data will be used. In this simple case, the requirement is to be able to identify who is waiting and their urgency.

Information will be needed:

- for the different waiting lists (codes and descriptions)
- to determine urgency (codes, descriptions and priority)
- to show details of patients' waiting list entries, including the status of the entries.

Data items will therefore include:

- a *Waiting List* code
- an *Urgency* code
- the *Date* a patient was put onto the list
- *Current status.*

5.9 Structuring data

Now that we have a feeling for the data items we need to collect, we will consider how they should be filed (structured). The structure of the data does not directly affect collection or retrieval, but it does affect how efficient the computer can be with both of these processes.

Computer storage is based around reducing duplication of storage, and developing a structure so that you can link related information together. The process for establishing a good storage structure for database information is called *data normalisation*.

5.9.1 Data normalisation

To arrive at a satisfactory computer data structure, we start with our data list and apply the four rules of data normalisation – which is mathematical 'set' theory applied to relational databases. These rules are discussed in the sections below.

You must first understand your data items. Below is the complete list; the items in italics have been obtained from the linked *patient.mdb* file – i.e. they do not need to be recollected.

- *Patient ID* – the computer-generated number used to identify patients
- *Patient UR Number* – the unique number used by the organisation's staff to identify the patient and their paper medical record
- *Surname*
- *Given Name*
- *Title*
- *Suffix*
- *Date of Birth*
- *Gender*
- Waiting List Code – for sorting and grouping entries
- Waiting List Description – full name of the waiting list, for reporting
- Urgency Code – for sorting and grouping
- Urgency Description – full name of the urgency category, for reporting
- Urgency Priority – numerical priority for sorting of entries
- Waiting List Status – status of patient's entry – still active or not
- Date patient put onto waiting list.

Computer efficiency requires a standardised approach to the representation of data. We call this representation an 'information model'. This model is a structure for the information that minimises duplication of data elements and assists in creating an efficient collection and storage system. Unfortunately, while this suits computers, for most people it is not the way a person would approach a similar problem. The process of developing the information model is called data normalisation and is represented by four 'normal forms', discussed below. The information model used in a simple database system such as Access is far less complex or versatile than those used more generally in information technology today. (For those interested in learning more, you might like to investigate UML modelling.)

The process, described below, starts with all your data fields and progressively considers how each element relates to the other elements in the data, in order to group elements with similar characteristics together and to build the model. The result will be a number of independent tables which can be linked together.

5.9.2   1st normal form

The first rule of normalisation is:

> group data in a way that ensures that data items do not repeat within the structure.

This is also called atomic form, because it can't be split any further. You are trying to ensure that any individual row in a table can't have more than one entry. A table is *not* in 1st normal form if any field can have multiple entries.

Figure 5.110 shows that an individual supervisor can have more than one person reporting to them – the People field contains multiple entries. Therefore, this sample is not in 1st normal form.

Department ID	Supervisor	People
1	3	Mary, Jayne, Sally, John
2	4	Allan, Wendy, Zara
3	9	Fiona, Bianca, Ruth

Figure 5.110 Sample table, *not* in 1st normal form

To work out what would be correct in 1st normal form, you need to look at and lift out multiple occurrences. In the example in Figure 5.110, each department only has a single supervisor. You could therefore have a table of departments and supervisors, which would be in 1st normal form. Now look at the people. Each person works in only one department, so you could have another table of people which indicates the department in which they work, which would also be in 1st normal form. You don't need to record the supervisor for each individual, as the two tables can be linked to provide this information.

EXERCISE 5.3 CONTINUED

In this section, instead of asking you to complete tasks, we will explain the process of normalising the data for this exercise. You should then complete the tasks in Exercise 5.4 on your own.

We already have a Patient Details table, outlined below, where the Patient ID field is a unique identifier – within the computer system – for each patient.

Patient Details
Patient ID
Patient UR Number
Surname
Given Name
Title
Suffix
Date of Birth
Gender
Nationality Code

It is important to note that the Patient UR Number can only be considered a unique ID *within the record-keeping system* – it is not the only unique identifier in the hospital or healthcare organisation that a person has (consider others such as Radiology Number or Pathology Number, or the local GP's filing number). The key for the Patient Details table must thus be the Patient ID, which is totally unique in the system and can be used to establish relationships between the Patient Details table and other tables in the database.

If you look at the list of data elements needed for this system, you will find other details not shown in the Patient Details table. Considering 1st normal form, we ask if a person can have more than one of any of these data elements. If a person can, then these elements must be in a separate table. For example:

- *Waiting List Code*
  Can a person be on more than one waiting list? Yes (therefore Waiting List Code should not be in Patient Details table).
- *Waiting List Description*
  Can a person have more than one waiting list description? Yes (therefore should not be in Patient Details table).
- *Urgency Code*
  Can a person have more than one urgency code? Yes (so, not in Patient Details table). And so on.

We now have two tables:

Patient Details	Patient Waiting List Entry
Patient ID	**Patient ID**
Patient UR Number	Waiting List Code
Surname	Waiting List Description
Given Name	Urgency Code
Title	Urgency Description
Suffix	Urgency Priority
Date of Birth	Waiting List Status
Gender	Date Patient put onto List
Nationality Code	

Consider the new table, and the potential relationships between these data elements. This is a waiting list for a person, therefore the Patient ID should be included in the table so that the link back to the patient as an individual is not lost.

Now consider what the second table contains. It is a description of an individual's entry on a waiting list (not a description of the individual). Considering 1st normal form, are there any items in this table that can occur more than once for an individual on the waiting list?

- They can be on more than one list, but that is not a problem, as we've already separated the patient from their potentially multiple entries on the waiting list.
- The individual's entry on any waiting list will have only one urgency at a time, and only one status at a time, and they will only be put on that list once.
- Problems arise in those data elements that don't actually relate *just* to this entry on the waiting list. These are the data elements that describe the

waiting list (such as the Waiting List Description) and the urgency (such as the Urgency Description and the Urgency Priority).

5.9.3 2nd normal form

Second normal form requires you to consider the key for each table:

within a table, all data items that are not part of the primary key must be dependent only upon the key data item(s).

What is the primary key for the Patient Waiting List Entry table? Think about what makes an entry in this table unique. To be unique, a primary key may include more than one data element, which together make the entry unique without restricting the functionality of the system.

In this case it is not the Patient ID alone, as choosing the Patient ID as the primary key would mean that the person can only *ever* be on the waiting list once, remembering that a primary key makes an entry unique. Can a person be on a particular waiting list more than once? Yes, but not at the same time. Therefore the key for the Patient Waiting List Entry table is the Patient ID *and* the Waiting List Code *and* the Date Patient put onto List.

Patient Waiting List Entry
Patient ID
Waiting List Code
Waiting List Description
Urgency Code
Urgency Description
Urgency Priority
Waiting List Status
Date Patient put onto List

When considering 2nd normal form, you need to establish that all of the data elements listed in this table are dependent upon the primary key. For example, is the Waiting List Description true for the Patient ID, the Waiting List Code and the Date Patient put onto List? No – it is true for the Waiting List Code irrespective of the patient involved or the date they were put onto the list. The proposed additional tables are:

Waiting List Codes
Waiting List Code
Waiting List Description

Urgency Codes
Urgency Code
Urgency Description
Urgency Priority

The tables show the keys in bold type – the keys are the data items that make the entry unique. The Patient Waiting List table is unique for a particular patient, placed on a particular waiting list at a specific time (this allows a person to be on a waiting list more than a single time).

This gives you a series of tables, in each of which data is linked to a single primary key (which may be made up of several parts).

In Exercise 5.3, look at the Patient Waiting List table, given below. Each patient's urgency will be specific to that patient, on that list, on that occasion (which correlates directly to the keys of Patient ID, Waiting List Code and Date on the waiting list.) In other words, the key to the patient's entry in the Patient Waiting List table are the data elements that will uniquely identify that person's entry on the list. Urgency and Waiting List Status 'belong' to that unique entry and therefore fit correctly in this table. This means that this table meets 2nd normal form rules.

Patient Waiting List
Patient ID **Waiting List Code** Urgency Code Waiting List Status **Date Patient put onto List**

5.9.4   3rd normal form

To normalise to 3rd normal form, you again look at the keys of each table:

the non-key fields are must be independent of all other non-key items.

Look again at the Patient Waiting List table above. It contains a Waiting List Status field and an Urgency Code field. These fields have no relationship to each other (they only relate to the primary key of patient/list/date). Therefore, the data structure meets 3rd normal form.

Table 5.4 Patient Waiting List table elements

Data item	Comments
Patient ID	To allow linkage to the Patient Details table
Waiting List Code	*Not* Waiting List Description because that would be repeated for every entry of this code. We create a new table to hold the waiting list codes and descriptions, and use the code to link from the Patient Waiting List table to the Waiting List Code table
Urgency Code	*Not* Urgency Description or Urgency Priority, again because there would be repetitions for each entry of a particular code. To reduce duplication, we create a separate table to reference these.
Waiting List Status	Whether the patient is waiting (Yes) or complete (No)
Date Patient put onto List	The date (dd/mm/yyyy) the patient was put on the waiting list

5.9.5 4th normal form

There also exists a 4th normal form, but it is rare that you would need to consider this; it usually relates only to very complex databases and is therefore not described here.

EXERCISE 5.4 (SELF-STUDY)

1 Create a new database with a suitable name, in a suitable folder/directory.

2 Link your new database to the one provided, *patients for recalls.mdb*.

3 Analyse what is required from the question to decide what data you need to collect.

4 Apply the rules of normalisation to your data fields to build a model for the structure of your data.

5 Confirm that you have a suitable data structure by referring to the completed example on the CD.

5.10 Reference and data tables

The database we are creating in Exercise 5.3 contains two different types of tables.

- The Patient Details table and the Patient Waiting List table hold details for individual people, real episode data, etc., and are called *data tables*.
- The Waiting List Codes table and the Urgency Codes table hold lists of valid codes and the descriptions and rules (priority) that apply to those codes. These are called *reference tables*.

You should build your reference tables first, as these will be used as automatic lookup tables (see section 5.10.1) by the data tables.

5.10.1 Reference tables

The data to be entered into these tables are given in Tables 5.5 and 5.6.

Table 5.5 Data for database Waiting List Code table

Waiting list code	Description
HR	Hip Replacement
CABG	Coronary Artery Bypass Graft
KR	Knee Replacement

Table 5.6 Data for database Urgency Code table

Urgency code	Description	Priority
U	To be admitted within 1 week	1
S	To be admitted within 1 month	2
R	To be admitted within 3 months	3
X	To be admitted without specified timeframe	4

EXERCISE 5.3 CONTINUED

4 Open your *WaitingList.mdb* database and choose to create a table in Design View. Use the data above to create the two reference tables **Waiting List Codes** and **Urgency Codes**. For each field you must enter:
   ❑ Field Name: the name you want to use for the data item.
   ❑ Data Type – can be Text (free text up to 255 characters long); Number (must be numeric); Date/Time (must be a date or time, or a combination of both); Memo (free text of unlimited size – but can't be sorted); others should be considered using Help if required.
   ❑ Description: describe the data item and its purpose.

As you enter each data item, the General tab in the Field Properties section allows you to enter specific rules for those data items, where appropriate. There are often few of these rules for reference tables.

Figure 5.111 shows the completed Waiting List Codes table. It is important to note that the field size specified for the Waiting List Code (which is a text field) is consistent with the size required for that field. Similar decisions on field format and size must be taken for every data item added to the table design.

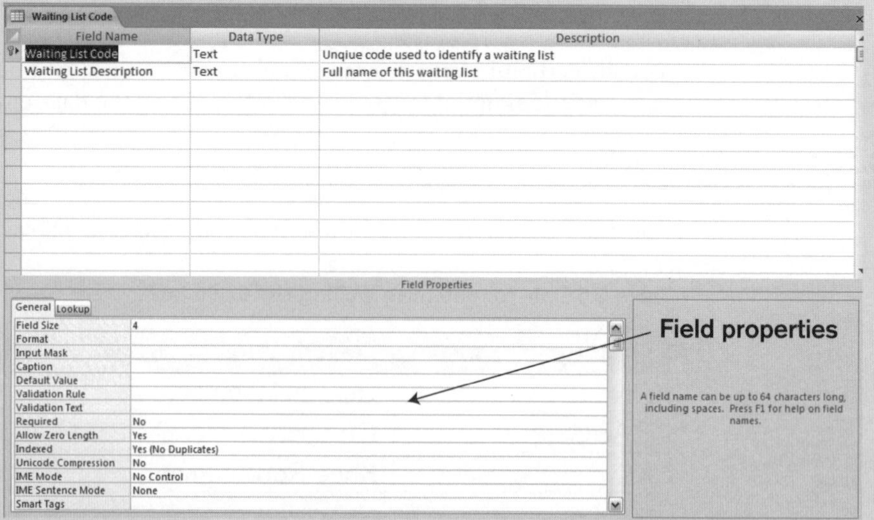

Figure 5.111
Waiting List
Code Table
in Design View

Remember to create an appropriate primary key for your each of your tables. If you forget and close or save the table, Access will ask you if you want to automatically create the key. Choose **No** and do it yourself, to make sure that it is appropriate for your needs. Check the tables outlined in section 5.9, where keys have been defined.

5   Once the tables are saved, go to Datasheet View and add the entries given in Tables 5.5 and 5.6.

5.10.2 Data tables and Lookup

The process for developing data tables is exactly the same as for reference tables, but there are some additional features you might use. The most common of these is the Lookup feature where you can have the system automatically look up reference tables to give you drop-down lists of possible code values. To create such a lookup, choose the Data Type to be Lookup Wizard.

EXERCISE 5.3 CONTINUED

6   Next we want to create our data tables. The Patient Details table is already there (it was the one we linked to), so we just need to create the Patient Waiting List table.
   ❑   With your *WaitingList.mdb* database open, choose to create a new table in Design View. Enter **Patient ID** as the first Field Name and choose the **Data Type** to be **Lookup Wizard** (Fig 5.112). This will open up the Lookup Wizard (Fig 5.113).

Figure 5.112
Starting the
Lookup
Wizard

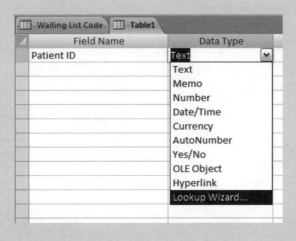

Figure 5.113
Initial Lookup
Wizard dialog
box

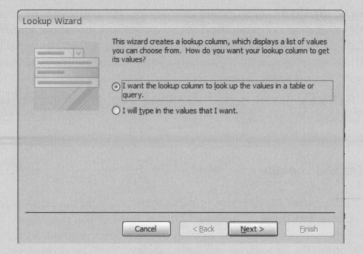

☐ You are using the wizard to look up details in an existing table (the default choice), so press **Next**. (You also have the option of entering specific data items to look up, rather than using a file in which to store those items.)

☐ Next, choose the table or query in which the codes/descriptions you need to look up are filed. To look up the patient details, choose the Patient Details table, and press **Next**.

☐ Now we need to select the data items (fields) we want to be looked up (Fig 5.114). For the Patient Waiting List table we want the Patient ID (as that is linked to the Patient Details table), Patient UR Number, Surname and Given Name (as these provide the information available to confirm the patient's ID).

Highlight each required item, and move it over to the **Selected Fields** area using the arrow keys. Remember that the sequence in which you select the data items will affect the way the system works. The computer will assume that the first field you choose is the one upon which the linkage will be created.

When you are ready, press **Next**.

Figure 5.114
Choosing the
field to be
looked up

Lookup Wizard

Which fields contain the values you want included in your lookup column? The fields you select become columns in your lookup column.

Available Fields:

| patient id |
| Patient UR number |
| surname |
| given name |
| title |
| Suffix |
| date of birth |
| gender |

Selected Fields:

Cancel   < Back   Next >   Finish

Next you are offered the ability to select one or more fields to sort the data by, so that it is easier for people to find the items they want off the list (Fig 5.115). You don't have to use this facility, but it can be helpful.

❏ Left-click on the down-arrow to see a list of possible fields for sorting. Selected Patient UR Number. (The system assumes you want to sort in an ascending order, so if you want descending order instead, click on the button to change it.) We do want ascending order, so press **Next**.

Figure 5.115
Sorting
records in the
Lookup
Wizard

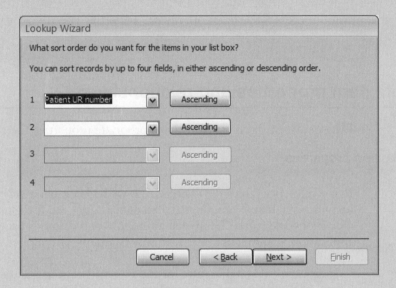

Figure 5.116, the next screen, shows how the lookup will appear in the final table. We have chosen to hide the actual key – the Patient ID is not a data field that users need to see or use; it is just a computer-related field.

❏ If you are happy with the layout, press **Next**.

Figure 5.116
Confirmation of
lookup fields

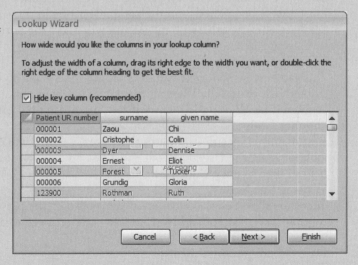

The last screen of the Lookup Wizard asks you to indicate the label for the lookup field; it defaults to the Patient ID we started with in our Waiting List table, so we will stick with that.

❐ Press **Finish**. You will be warned that you need to save the table in order to create a relationship link between the tables (the one you are building and the Patient Details table you are looking up from). Choose **Yes** and name your table **Patient Waiting List**. Choose not to set a primary key at this stage.

We will now move on to discuss data item (field) properties before completing the rest of this table.

5.11 Data item properties and relationships

Data items (fields) must have the appropriate properties and relationships.

5.11.1 Data item properties

In the reference tables for Exercise 5.3, we had comparatively simple data items to establish. The more detailed data designs require more complex definitions and rules. Before you attempt to enforce rules using the database application, you must have a clear understanding of the rules you need to introduce.

Indications of suitable rules for the Patient Waiting List table are given below. We will then work through the stages of how to establish these rules. The Patient Waiting List table file requires the following data items:

- **Patient ID**
  This can best be managed by a direct link to the Patient Details table through a lookup (as we have already done). The Patient ID is a field that must always be entered; and the patient must be in the Patient Details database already, otherwise the system will reject the entry (you can't have a Waiting List entry if there is no patient specified).
- **Waiting List Code**
  This can best be managed by a direct link to the Waiting List Codes table through a lookup. The Waiting List Code is a field that must be entered, as there is no Waiting List entry if the patient isn't put onto a waiting list.
- **Urgency Code**
  Best managed by a direct link to the Urgency Codes table through a lookup; again the Urgency Code must be entered, and it must be a code held in the Urgency Code table.
- **Waiting List Status**
  This should be Yes or No, where Yes means that the person is still waiting for treatment and No that they have received treatment or no longer require treatment.
- **Date patient put onto the list**
  This should be a date field, which could default to 'today's date' as data

entry would normally be done directly at the time the request to join a waiting list was processed. A *default* fills in the field automatically, but can be changed. This date should not be able to be a future date, as that would be illogical.

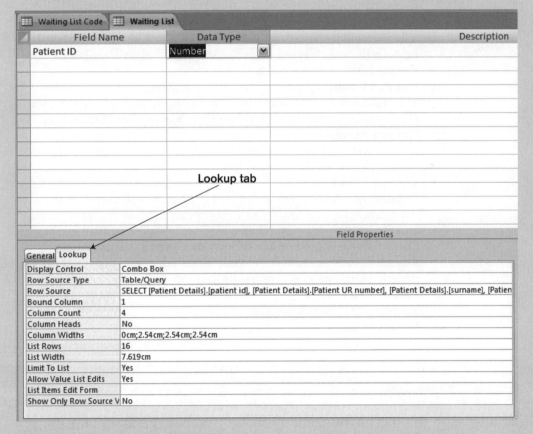
The Lookup tab shows the details established by your choices using the Lookup Wizard. The controls include:

- **Display Control**
  A Combo Box lists the options available for selection, and is the most common choice for shorter drop-down lists. It also restricts you to selecting only one of the items that is in the list.
    Go to Datasheet View for an open table, and see how this works. You should make alternative choices in Design View, and go back to Datasheet View to see how they change the display of data options.
- **Row Source Type**
  Indicates what type of source the data is coming from; this could be a table or query, a list of values you enter yourself, or a list of fields. When you use the Lookup Wizard, these details are automatically entered with the right syntax.
- **Row Source**
  Indicates the actual source of the lookup data, in this case [table name]. [field name], [table name], [next field name], etc. (Square brackets are used where a table name or field name is more than one word.) Sort details are also included.
- **Bound Column**
  This indicates which column in the table being looked up contains the field that will be placed in the Patient Waiting List table's Patient ID field. In this case it is the first column of the Patient Details table (the Patient ID).
- **Column Count**
  This indicates the number of fields to be shown in the lookup on screen (in this case, fields Patient UR Number, Surname and Given Name).
- **Column Headings**
  Do you want to show the column headings in the lookup? No is the normal choice for drop-down lists.
- **Column Width**
  Details the display width for each of the columns displayed in the drop-down list.
- **List Rows**
  Gives the maximum number of rows that will be displayed in the drop-down list. If there are more records in the table than this number, a scroll bar will be shown as part of the drop-down box.
- **Line Width**
  Width of the drop-down box.
- **Limit to List**
  This can be set to Yes or No.

EXERCISE 5.3 CONTINUED

8 In our case, our requirement that the patients must be in the Patient Details table means that we must set the Limit to List to Yes.
    If you are unsure how this works, try changing the value and then entering data that is not already in the Patient Details table.

The other requirement for the Patient ID is that it needs to be a mandatory field – it *must* be entered. To control this, go to the **General** tab in Design View while having the Patient ID data type selected (Fig 5.118).

Figure 5.118
General tab layout

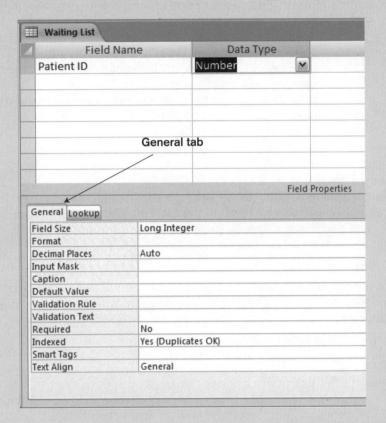

Again, the values in these fields were established automatically when we used the Lookup Wizard to define the field. Changes should thus not be made to Field Size, Format, Decimal Places or Input Mask.

❏ We want to make sure the Patient ID is always entered. To do this, set the value in box next to **Required** to **Yes**.

❏ Choosing Yes for the property **Indexed** makes searching and sorting more efficient. The default entry here, **Yes (Duplicates OK)**, indicates that the system will allow a patient to have more than one entry in the table, but that this is a field that has been indexed for fast retrieval.

9 Continue to build the Patient Waiting List table in a similar way, making sure that your system meets the requirements listed previously for the fields Waiting List Code and Urgency Code and Waiting List Status. Check that you have got what you want by entering data in Datasheet View.

10 Now we get to the field 'Date patient put onto the list'. The date properties are more complex.

❑ First, choose the Data Type of **Date/Time**. Now go to the **General** tab and look at the range of choices for **Format**, which will be shown along with examples something like these:

General Date	19/06/1998 5:34:03 PM
Long Date	Sunday, 19 June 1998
Medium Date	19-Jun-98
Short Date	19/06/1998 (the most common format used)
Long Time	5:34:03 PM
Medium Time	5:34 PM
Short Time	17:34

Short Date is fine for this field.

❑ Next, we want the date to default to 'today's date'. This is done by using the special instruction **Now()** in the **Default Value** box. The brackets () tell Access that this is a special program word.

Quick hint

There are many other special program words (we will look at some of them in more detail in the Build option). Common expressions you may find useful are:

- Now() – inserts today's date/time
- Today() – inserts today without reference to time
- Null() – meaning empty.

There is an expression builder which you may choose to investigate further, but the functionality is not described in this introductory text.

❑ The next step is to establish a rule that forbids future dates – for this you use the **Validation Rule** box. Type in **<=Now()** to add the rule that the date entered must be less than or equal to 'today's date'.

If this rule is not met by the date entered, the user will be shown an error message. If you don't enter a specific message in the **Validation Message** box, the program will generate a message. It is always better for you to enter a message that users will understand rather than leave it to the program. Type in **You cannot enter a future date**.

❑ Finally, ensure that there is a **Yes** in the **Required** box. If you have already entered data into your fields, you may get a message warning that data integrity rules may be broken by this change. If there is no data in the system, accepting this is okay (this is the reason for setting this up before entering data).

Figure 5.119 shows the final list of General field properties.

Figure 5.119
General properties for the field 'Date patient put onto the list'

Waiting List Code	Waiting List		
Field Name	**Data Type**		
Patient ID	Number	Unique identifier t
Waiting List code	Text	The waiting list ind
Urgency Code	Text	The urgency with w
Waiting List Status	Yes/No	YES indicatesthat tl
Date patient put onto the wait	Date/Time	⌄	

Field Properties

General | Lookup

Format	Short Date
Input Mask	
Caption	
Default Value	Now()
Validation Rule	>=Now()
Validation Text	You cannot enter a future date
Required	Yes ⌄
Indexed	No
IME Mode	No Control
IME Sentence Mode	None
Smart Tags	
Text Align	General
Show Date Picker	For dates

Quick hint

You can also use the Validation Rule box to hold a short set of options for a field. These will not show as a drop-down list, but will restrict the data that can be entered.

For example, if you wanted only the values M or F to be accepted for a Sex field, you would enter **M or F** into the Validation Rule box. The computer would change the layout of your entry to 'M' or 'F' and would insist that the values entered in this field meet this requirement.

11 Make sure that each field has a description that makes clear what the intent of the data item is. In this way, if you come back to the design some months or years later you will be able to remember what you intended. This also makes it much easier for another staff member who might take over after you leave your job to understand what the database is about.

When all the data items are completed, create a primary key for this table.

Before, we have always been able to pick a single field (row) to make the primary key, but this table is a bit different. Remember that the keys is what make a single record in the table unique. In our Patient Waiting List table, what makes a record unique is the Patient ID combined with the Waiting List Code and with Date patient put onto list.

Look at Figure 5.120 – multiple rows have been set to be the key.

❑ To do this, highlight the whole of the first row by left-clicking in the small shaded column to the left, Then hold down the **CTRL** key while you highlight the additional row. Now right-click and select **Primary key**.

Field Name	Data Type	Description
🔑 Patient ID	Number	Unique identifier that links tables together
🔑 Waiting List code	Text	The waiting list indicating the procedure for which the persc
Urgency Code	Text	The urgency with which this person must be given treatmen
Waiting List Status	Yes/No	YES indicatesthat the person is still waiting while NO indicat
🔑▶ Date patient put onto the wait	Date/Time	

Tabs: Waiting List Code | Waiting List

Figure 5.120 Patient Waiting List table in Design View, showing key selection

5.11.2 Relationships

Using the Lookup Wizard will have established certain relationships between our Exercise 5.3 tables. These should be checked and the data model reviewed.

EXERCISE 5.3 CONTINUED

12 First, close all Design View windows. To open the Relationships window:
   ❑ in Access 2007, go to **Database Tools ➤ Relationships**
   ❑ in Access 2003, go to **Tools ➤ Relationships** or press the Relationships icon in the toolbar (Fig 5.121).

This icon is only active when you have no Design View windows open.

Figure 5.121 Relationships icon

When the **Relationships** window first opens, the tables will be shown in a row, which may obscure some of the relationships. Drag the tables around until they form a logical and clean representation. You may also want to resize some of the table boxes to show all the data items properly.

Figure 5.122 shows the correct relationships required to support the *WaitingList.mdb* database.

Figure 5.122
Relationships
for *WaitingList.
mdb* database

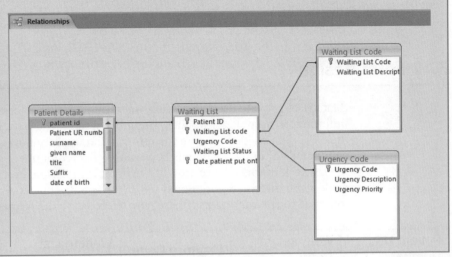

EXERCISE 5.4 (SELF-STUDY) CONTINUED

Quick hint

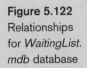

If you accidentally
create a relationship
that is not what you
intended, select
the relationship line
(which will make it
darker), then right-
click and choose
delete.

For the recall letters, you have patient information and
you have information about the letters to be sent. Your
data structure should reflect the following data needs:

Patient Details   *Follow Up*

                           Patient ID

                           Letter Type

                           Letter Name

                           Date Letter to be Sent

                           Letter Sent

6   Using the data structure you have determined and confirmed, list the
requirements for each data item in each table you need to create. You are likely
to need a reference table for Letter Type and Letter Name.

7   Create all the tables and set the Field Properties as required. Date properties
for Date Letter to be Sent should be considered.

8   Check the relationships between your tables to see if they are what you
identified as being required.

9   Check the Field properties of each data item, and the relationships between
tables, against the completed example on the CD.

Once tables have been established for a database, a screen can be designed that can be used to collect the information needed. These screens are called *forms*.

5.12 Form design

Databases provide features to help you design screens – forms – for collecting information accurately. In our waiting list system, you have identified the fields of data needed to store the information, and are now ready to actually add details of individuals and their waiting list requirements to the system.

The task in this next section of the book is to design a form you can use to collect the information required for Exercise 5.3. This requires us to add new referrals to the waiting list; these new referrals are the four entries below.

Patient UR Number	Waiting List Code	Urgency Code	Waiting List Status	Date put onto list
676883	HR	X	Yes	10 Jan 2009
134141	CABG	R	Yes	10 Apr 2008
194882	KR	S	Yes	28 Sep 2008
300233	CABG	U	Yes	10 Jan 2008

The forms creation facility is what allows you to simply design a form that helps with data entry. You can choose the fields to be included on the form, and the way that those fields will look. We will start by introducing the concepts via the Form Wizard.

5.12.1 Form Wizard

The Form Wizard guides you through the process of designing a form, and is what you should use unless you are *very* familiar with form design.

EXERCISE 5.3 CONTINUED

13 Open your database *WaitingList.mdb*.
  ❐ In Access 2007, go to **Create ➤ Form**.
  ❐ In Access 2003, select the **Forms** section of the main database window and choose **Create form by using Wizard**.

This will bring up the first dialog box of the Form Wizard, shown in Figure 5.123, with the first (alphabetical) table or query visible.
  ❐ Select **Patient Waiting List** as the table/query to form the basis of the form.
  ❐ Now, in a similar way to the Report Wizard, the fields in that table will be visible in the **Available Fields** section. Select the fields you want, in the order you want those fields to appear on the form.

Figure 5.123
Form Wizard
– select table
and data
items

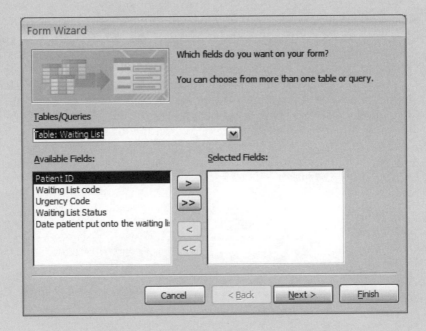

Figure 5.124 shows a list of selections for the waiting list entry form. Take note of the sequence, as this will be reflected in the final format. When you are happy with your choices, press **Next**.

Figure 5.124
Form Wizard
showing
selected field
choices

Next, choose the layout style for your form (Fig 5.125). The layout style affects both the way the form works and the look of the form. A Columnar format will present data in columns, one record at a time. The Tabular format will show each record in a table, and a Datasheet will be similar (but look like a Datasheet). Like Columnar format, Justified shows one record at a time. The sample shown here is a Justified form.

❑ Choose **Justified** style, and press **Next**.

Figure 5.125
Form Wizard –
layout style

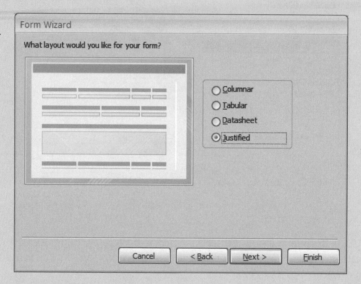

❑ Now you are offered different options for the way the final form will look (Fig 5.126). Standard is a good, clean option! Choose something appropriate and press **Next**.

Figure 5.126
Form Wizard
– choosing a
look

❑ Finally, you are asked to give your form a title (Fig 5.127). The name of the table from which you started will appear at the top of the screen as the form name.

We recommend that you don't change the automatic suggestion of opening the form to view or enter information, as it is best to check that the form looks as you expected it to.

❑ Press **Finish**. Figure 5.128 shows the result.

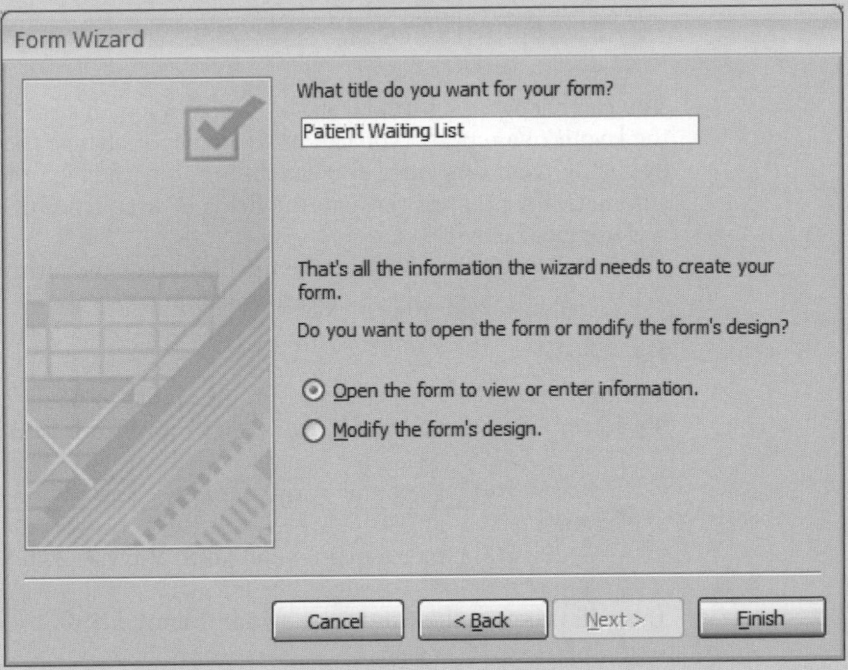

Figure 5.127
Form Wizard
– final window

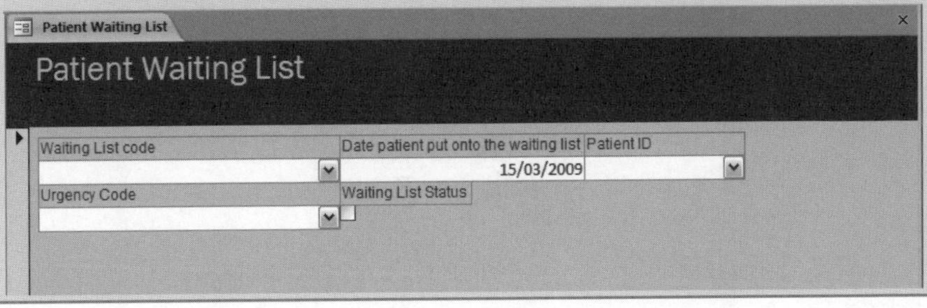

Figure 5.128
Final form for
data entry
created using
Form Wizard

5.12.2 Form in Design View

To tidy up the design of the form we have created in Exercise 5.3, go to Design View (Fig 5.129).

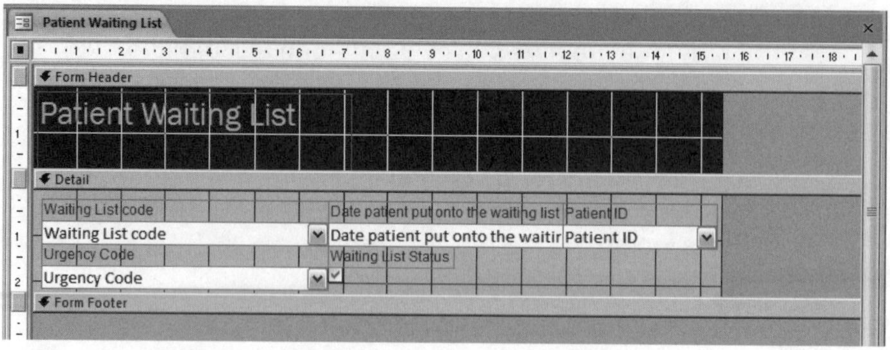

Figure 5.129
Form in Design
View

You can change the form layout in Design View in a similar way to changing the layout of a report – you can move items, or change their size and shape, by clicking and dragging. You can also modify the tab order so that you automatically progress through the fields in a sequence that suits your design and use (see below).

We will return to adjusting the final layout of the form after section 5.12.4; do not make any changes at this point.

Tab order

This option for form layout gives you the ability to modify the sequence of the cursor when you press the Tab key to move from field to field.

- In Access 2007, go to the **Forms Design Tools** ribbon and choose the **Arrange** tab.
- In Access 2003, in the main menu go to **View ➤ Tab Order**.

This will bring up the window shown in Figure 5.130.

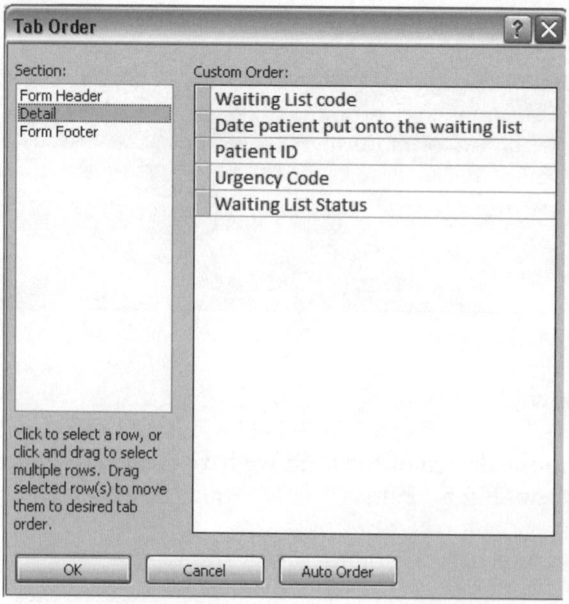

Figure 5.130
Changing tab
order for a form

This screen allows you to modify the tab order in the Form Header, Detail and Form Footer sections. (Our form currently only has fields in the Detail section.)

The tab order will default to the same sequence as you had when you initially selected the data items. To change this order, select an item on the list (it will become highlighted when you click on the box next to the name) and drag the item to the place on the list where you would like it to appear in the tab sequence. This will not change the order of items on the screen, only the order in which the cursor visits those item for data entry.

5.12.3 Subform

The form we have now created for entering waiting list data includes a lot of repetition. For example, the Waiting List Code is repeated in every line. It would look better – and be more efficient in terms of data entry – if the Waiting List Code appeared at the top of the form and the details for each patient were then entered below. This concept is outlined below.

Waiting List: Knee Replacement			
Date On List	Patient Number	Urgency	Status
14/1/08	191802	S	
20/1/08	778221	U	
13/1/09	661224	S	Done

Forms designed like this *can* be produced, but they require the system to produce two forms: one at the level of the Patient Waiting List table, and one at the level of the individual patient entry details for that waiting list. This two-part form (heading and subsection) is called a subform.

Creating a subform
The process of creating a subform is similar to that of a basic form, but there are some additional choices to make in the Form Wizard that will confirm that you are achieving a multipart form.

EXERCISE 5.3 CONTINUED

14 Begin by starting the Form Wizard for a new form.
- ❒ Now, select the **Waiting List Codes** table and then **Waiting List Code** and **Waiting List Description** from the list of available fields.
- ❒ Then change the table to **Patient Waiting List**, and select the additional fields you want in the lower section of the form: **Date put on list, Patient ID, Urgency Code** and **Waiting List Status**. Figure 5.131 shows the final choice of fields from the two tables. The sequence of fields selected will still affect the way the final form/subform looks.
- ❒ When your selections are complete, press **Next**.

Figure 5.131
Field
selection for a
multipart form

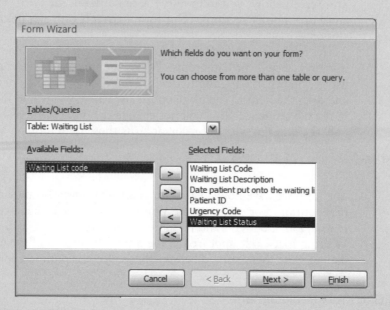

Figure 5.132 shows the result. This is a window that did not appear during the simpler form design process. It shows that the Waiting List Codes table is the 'base' form and the Patient Details table supplies the subform. The base form should always be the area you want at the top of the form – the data that occurs once per display – while the subform usually represents multiple records for each single base form.

Figure 5.132
Form and
subform
creation

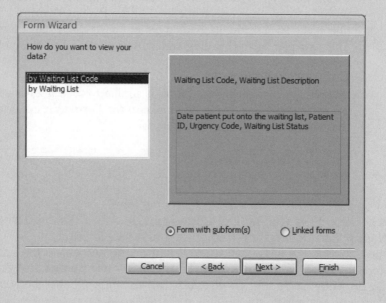

You can also use linked forms, which open a separate window from the base form. Figure 5.133 shows the choice of linked forms.

Figure 5.133
Linked forms
selection

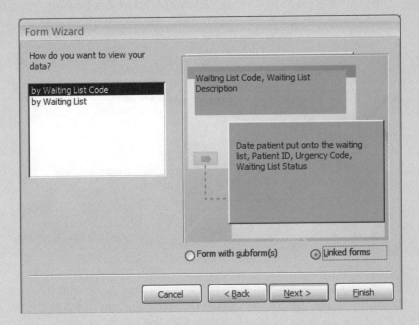

☐ For Exercise 5.3, choose **Form with subform(s)** as this is the most appropriate style. Press **Next.**

We can now choose the layout for the subform. You are offered two choices – Tabular or Datasheet; these are fairly similar and your choice will not greatly affect the operation of the form, simply its look and feel.

Figure 5.134
Subform
layout
selection

- ☐ Select **Tabular** style and press **Next**. Choose a suitable style in the next window, and press **Next** again.
- ☐ The final step is similar to that for a simple form, but this time you are saving *two* form designs: the base form and the subform (Fig 5.135). Choose suitable names, and press **Finish** to open the form to view or enter information.

Figure 5.135
Saving the
multipart form
design

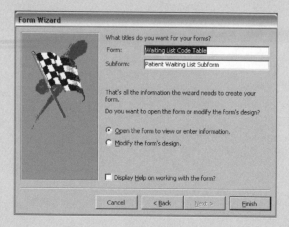

Figure 5.136 shows the final multipart form produced. Note that there are now two record movement bars on the window: one at the bottom of the subform and one at the bottom of the base form. The movement is the same for each.

Figure 5.136
Final design
of a form with a
subform:
(top) Design
View;
(bottom)
ready to enter
data

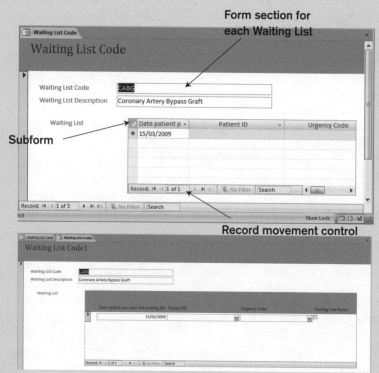

When you save the form, two forms are actually created. Figure 5.137 shows the forms now saved.

Figure 5.137
Saved subform

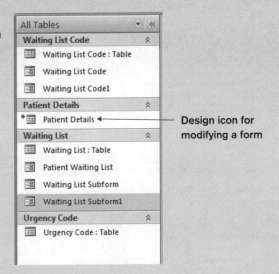

Design icon for modifying a form

The form is saved with the name you gave it, and the subform has a name indicating that it is a subform.

To make changes to the *design*, you can choose either the form or subform and open in Design View. To add (enter) data you should always choose the form (not the subform). If you enter data just in a subform, the relationships to other data items will not be maintained. For example, you wouldn't have a waiting list specified for a new patient being added to that waiting list.

5.12.4 Design changes to subforms and forms

The detailed look of a form can be changed in Design View in a similar way to reports (see section 5.5.2)

Exercise 5.3 continued

15 Open your multipart form in Form View (this is what you get if you double-click on the form in the Forms section of the main database window, and is the equivalent of Datasheet View for a table or query). Review the form (Fig 5.136). Are there any elements of the design that could be improved? Yes:
  ❐ The subform needs more space to show the waiting list status.
  ❐ The form could show the waiting list description next to the code. The full headings for the code and description are not really needed, so that area of the design could be changed.
  ❐ You could show more patient entries if the subform was larger.

16 Now go to Design View (Fig 5.138).

Figure 5.138
Design View
of form and
subform

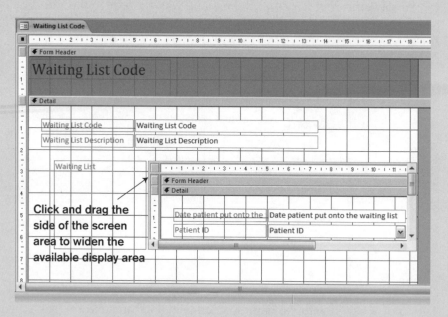

The first step is to make the display area wider. Figure 5.138 shows where to extend the design area, and Figure 5.139 shows the result of this. Note that there is still more space at the right side of the form area after the move.

Figure 5.139
Result of
widening the
space of the
view

17 The properties of the 'Date patient put onto the waiting list' field can be modified to allow the field to grow (in the same way as done in the Report section).

❑ Go to Form View in the Datasheet style version, and click and drag the size of the column until it is large enough to show all the date heading. An alternative way is to (right-click) open the Properties box for an item (similar to how it is done in reports), and select **Grow**. This will size the item according to the content of what is entered.

❑ Go back to Design View and modify the other headings so that they are appropriate to the space and requirements of the user. The design result is shown in Figure 5.140. Check your changes in Datasheet View.

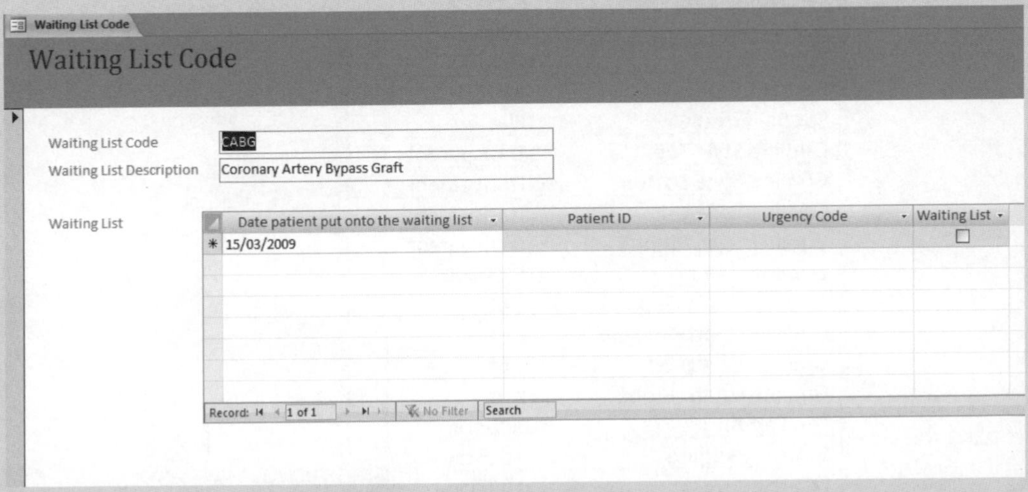

Figure 5.140 Display of modified data structure

18 You may find that some changes you make to the heading in the Form Header section don't show when you go to Form View. If this is the case, it will be because you chose a Datasheet style for the design layout of the Subform.

❑ Datasheets always show the field name at the top of the column. To change the design layout, open the Subform (rather than the main form) in Design View, then right-click and choose **Properties**. This will bring up the form's properties window (Fig 5.141). (In Access 2007, the Home ribbon included the Properties Sheet icon on the far right when you are in Design View.)

Figure 5.141
Form
Properties.
Note the
drop-down
box for the
form title,
which allows
you to easily
review
properties for
other parts of
the form

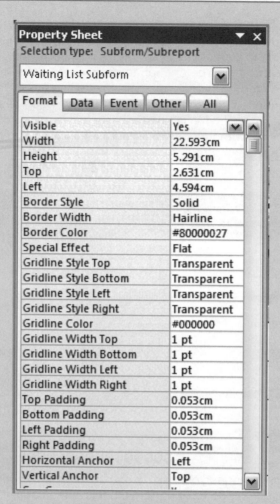

Property Sheet	▼ ✕
Selection type: Subform/Subreport	

Waiting List Subform ⌄

| Format | Data | Event | Other | All |

Visible	Yes ⌄
Width	22.593cm
Height	5.291cm
Top	2.631cm
Left	4.594cm
Border Style	Solid
Border Width	Hairline
Border Color	#80000027
Special Effect	Flat
Gridline Style Top	Transparent
Gridline Style Bottom	Transparent
Gridline Style Left	Transparent
Gridline Style Right	Transparent
Gridline Color	#000000
Gridline Width Top	1 pt
Gridline Width Bottom	1 pt
Gridline Width Left	1 pt
Gridline Width Right	1 pt
Top Padding	0.053cm
Bottom Padding	0.053cm
Left Padding	0.053cm
Right Padding	0.053cm
Horizontal Anchor	Left
Vertical Anchor	Top

❐ Under the **All** tab, change **Default View** to **Continuous forms** – and your heading change will take effect. The look of this change and the changes indicated in the next two figures are shown in Figure 5.144.

19 To make more space for the Subform, you need to increase the space allocated on the base form for display of the Subform. Open the base form in the Design View and left-click on the Subform space. Figure 5.142 shows the design of the Subform area, while Figure 5.143 shows that the Subform design area can be changed in the same way as the Form area of the base form.

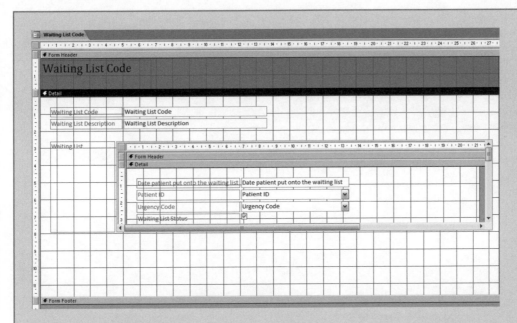

Figure 5.142 Base form before resizing

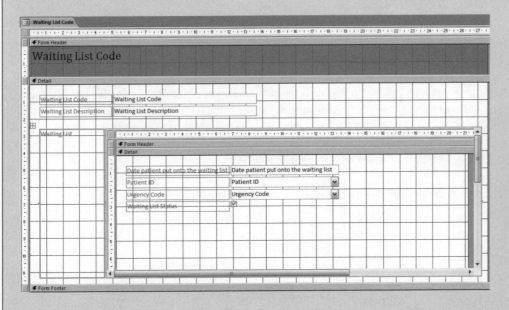

Figure 5.143 Resized Subform space in the base form

The results of these changes are shown in Figure 5.144 (Form View).

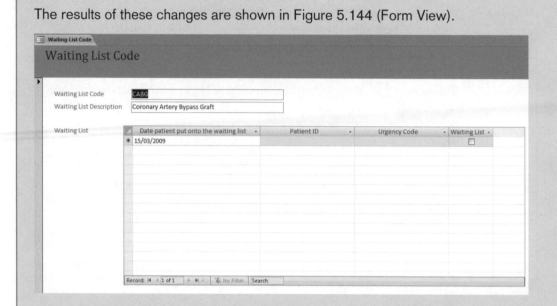

Figure 5.144 Final screen layout

---

10 Create a form to collect data, and try producing reports from the data collected. In the previous section, you created a file structure to hold details of the follow-up requirements. You will need to make sure that you have entered the letter types and codes into the Letter table before you enter patient details. The letters to be sent and the codes are given below.

Letter to be sent	Patient Number	Letter type	Status
14/1/2009	223344	Pap smear	
20/1/2009	778822	Visit	
13/1/2010	553322	Tetanus	

Letter types	Code
Pap smear	PS
Visit	V
Tetanus	TT
Inoculation	IN

5.12.5 Troubleshooting forms

The most common problems with forms derive from inappropriate data table design or relationships.

For example, if you are designing a form, and expect a Subform to be shown in the screen layout part of the Form Wizard process – but it is not, this means that the tables from which you chose your fields on the form have a one-to-one relationship. Subforms are only offered when the data selected for inclusion in the form are from tables that have a one-to-many relationship.

Problems can also be experienced if you have established a relationship between a data item that has a specific structure in the first table and a different structure in the Subform table. For example: the Waiting List Codes table has the Waiting List Code structured as text four digits long, while in the Patient Waiting List table the Waiting List Code is structured as text two digits long. A relationship between the two will not work, because relationships must be between items that are exactly the same in format.

5.13 Summary

Databases are a powerful tool, providing the capacity to manipulate data without the need for detailed programming skills. Although the examples given here are in some cases quite complex, there are cases where a simple report can be produced quickly and simply from a data collection.

Review questions

1 What are some of the tasks for which a database is particularly useful?

2 When asking for data to be extracted for your use, what important information do you need to provide to the person providing you with the data?

3 When designing a report, what are some of the design components you need to consider? (Think about the content – what fields?, the sequence of data, selection criteria, etc.) Why are these so important?

Index